INTRODUCTION

Myasthenia Gravis (MG) is a rare and chronic autoimmune neuromuscular disorder that affects the communication between nerves and muscles. In individuals with MG, the immune system mistakenly attacks and weakens the receptors responsible for transmitting nerve signals to muscles. This results in muscle weakness, particularly in the voluntary muscles that control facial expressions, eye movements, swallowing, and limb movements. Fluctuating symptoms, with periods of exacerbation and remission, characterize MG.

The hallmark feature of MG is muscle fatigability, where strength diminishes with prolonged activity and improves with rest. This condition can impact various aspects of daily life, leading to challenges in speaking, chewing, lifting objects, and maintaining physical endurance.

A well-considered eating plan can play a supportive role in managing symptoms and promoting overall health. Individuals with MG often face difficulties related to muscle weakness and fatigue, and the potential side effects of medications further emphasize the importance of a thoughtful dietary approach.

Critical considerations for a Myasthenia Gravis diet include:

1. Balanced Nutrition: Emphasize a balanced diet rich in fruits, vegetables, whole grains, lean proteins, and healthy fats. A diverse range of nutrients supports overall well-being.

2. Small, Frequent Meals: Consuming more minor, more frequent meals helps manage fatigue and prevents excessive energy expenditure during digestion, minimizing the impact on weakened muscles.

3. Hydration: Adequate hydration is crucial, especially if swallowing difficulties are present. Regular intake of water and hydrating fluids is essential to prevent dehydration.

4. Protein-Rich Foods: Include sources of lean protein, such as poultry, fish, tofu, and legumes, to support muscle health and aid in repair.

5. Identification of Trigger Foods: Some individuals may experience symptom exacerbation after consuming specific foods. Identifying and avoiding potential trigger foods can be beneficial, though this varies among individuals.

6. Supplementation: Depending on individual needs and medication interactions, supplementation of vitamins and minerals, including calcium and vitamin D, may be recommended for overall health.

This isn't just a diet; it's a personalized gastronomic adventure, an exploration of flavors that cater to the unique palate of an individual living with MG. It's about savoring the joy of a well-prepared meal that fuels the body and ignites a sense of vitality and strength.

CHAPTER ONE

Understanding Myasthenia Gravis

Myasthenia Gravis (MG) is a rare and chronic autoimmune neuromuscular disorder characterized by muscle weakness and fatigue. In this intricate condition, the immune system mistakenly targets and attacks the acetylcholine receptors (AChR) at the neuromuscular junction, where nerves communicate with muscles. The result is impaired communication between nerve and muscle cells, leading to weakness, especially in the voluntary muscles.

CAUSES AND RISK FACTORS OF MYASTHENIA GRAVIS

Myasthenia Gravis (MG) is an autoimmune disorder characterized by muscle weakness, and its origins lie in a complex interplay of genetic, immunological, and environmental factors. While the precise cause of MG remains elusive, a nuanced understanding of its potential triggers and associated risk factors provides valuable insights into the multifaceted nature of this condition.

1. Autoimmune Dysfunction:

• Primary Cause: MG is fundamentally an autoimmune disorder where the immune system, responsible for defending the body against foreign invaders, erroneously targets and attacks components of the neuromuscular junction—specifically, the acetylcholine receptors (AChR) or other proteins essential for nerve-muscle communication.

• Antibody-Mediated: In a majority of MG cases, the immune system produces antibodies that block or destroy AChR, disrupting the transmission of nerve signals to muscles.

2. Genetic Predisposition:

• Familial Occurrence: While MG is not directly inherited, there is evidence of a genetic predisposition. Individuals with a family history of autoimmune disorders may have a higher risk of developing MG.

3. Thymus Abnormalities:

• Association with Thymus: The thymus gland, a vital component of the immune system located in the chest, is often implicated in MG. Thymic abnormalities, including thymomas (tumors) or hyperplasia (enlargement), are found in a significant proportion of individuals with MG.

• Thymectomy Impact: Surgical removal of the thymus (thymectomy) can sometimes lead to symptom improvement, reinforcing the link between MG and thymus abnormalities.

4. Immunological Triggers:

• Viral Infections: Certain viral infections, including respiratory and gastrointestinal viruses, have been suggested as potential triggers for MG. These infections may stimulate an autoimmune response in susceptible individuals.

5. Hormonal Influence:

• Hormonal Changes: MG is known to be more prevalent in women and often emerges during periods of hormonal fluctuations, such as puberty, pregnancy, or menopause. Hormonal factors may contribute to the modulation of the immune response.

6. Medications:

• Medication-Induced MG: Some medications, such as certain antibiotics and muscle relaxants, may trigger symptoms resembling MG. However, discontinuing these medications often leads to symptom resolution.

7. Age and Gender:

• Age and Gender Prevalence: MG can affect individuals of any age, but it is more common in young adult women and older men. Juvenile Myasthenia Gravis specifically affects children and adolescents.

8. Other Autoimmune Conditions:

• Overlap with Autoimmune Disorders: Individuals with MG may have a higher likelihood of having or developing other autoimmune disorders, suggesting a shared immunological basis.

MYASTHENIA GRAVIS SYMPTOMS

Myasthenia Gravis (MG) is a complex neuromuscular disorder characterized by a diverse array of symptoms stemming from the disruption of communication between nerves and muscles. The clinical presentation of MG is often distinctive, marked by muscle weakness that can affect various parts of the body. Understanding the breadth and variability of these symptoms is crucial for timely diagnosis and effective management.

1. Muscle Weakness:

• Fatigability: A hallmark feature of MG is muscle weakness that intensifies with activity and improves with rest. This fatigue is particularly noticeable during repetitive movements or sustained muscle use.

2. Ocular Symptoms:

• Ptosis: Drooping of one or both eyelids, known as ptosis, is a common early symptom of MG. It can affect the vision and may fluctuate throughout the day.

• Double Vision (Diplopia): Weakness in the eye muscles can result in double vision, where a single object appears as two separate images.

3. Facial and Neck Muscles:

• Facial Weakness: Weakness in the facial muscles may lead to difficulty in smiling, frowning, or maintaining facial expressions.

• Difficulty Swallowing (Dysphagia): Impaired muscle function in the throat and neck can cause difficulty in swallowing, leading to choking or coughing while eating or drinking.

4. Limb Weakness:

• Proximal Muscle Weakness: MG can affect the muscles closer to the body's core, resulting in arm and leg weakness. Climbing stairs or lifting objects may become challenging.

5. Respiratory Involvement:

• Breathing Difficulties: In severe cases, MG can impact the respiratory muscles, leading to shortness of breath and respiratory distress. This is a medical emergency requiring immediate attention.

6. Voice Changes:

• Hoarseness: Weakness in the muscles controlling the vocal cords can lead to a hoarse or whispery voice.

7. Fluctuating Symptoms:

• Variable Presentation: MG symptoms can vary in intensity and may come and go. Individuals may experience periods of exacerbation followed by periods of relative improvement.

8. Exacerbating Factors:

• Aggravation with Activity: Symptoms often worsen with physical activity and improve with rest. Restoring strength after a period of rest is a characteristic feature.

9. Time of Day Influence:

• Worsening in the Evening: Many individuals with MG report increased weakness in the evening, reflecting the cumulative impact of daily activities.

10. Generalized Weakness:

• Overall Fatigue: Beyond muscle-specific weakness, individuals with MG may experience general fatigue and a sense of exhaustion.

DIAGNOSTIC OF MYASTHENIA GRAVIS

Diagnosing Myasthenia Gravis (MG) involves a meticulous blend of clinical evaluation, neurological examination, and specialized tests aimed at unraveling the intricate neuromuscular dynamics. Here is the diagnostic process:

A. Clinical Evaluation:

• Patient History: The journey begins with a thorough exploration of the patient's medical history, paying close attention to the onset and progression of symptoms. Any family history of autoimmune disorders or thymic abnormalities is noted.

• Symptom Analysis: A detailed discussion focuses on the nature and patterns of muscle weakness, fluctuation of symptoms, and any exacerbating or alleviating factors.

B. Neurological Examination:

• Ocular Assessment: A critical component involves examining ocular muscles for signs of ptosis (drooping eyelids) and diplopia (double vision).

• Facial and Bulbar Muscles: Evaluation extends to

facial expressions, speech, and swallowing, probing for weakness or difficulty in these areas.

• Limb Strength Assessment: Proximal limb muscle weakness is assessed through tasks like rising from a chair or lifting the arms.

C. Electromyography (EMG):

• Objective Neuromuscular Assessment: EMG is a pivotal diagnostic tool that provides objective evidence of neuromuscular dysfunction. It involves the insertion of fine needles into specific muscles to record electrical activity. In MG, abnormal patterns, such as rapid fatigue during repetitive stimulation, may be observed.

D. Blood Tests for Antibodies:

• Detection of Antibodies: Blood tests are conducted to identify specific antibodies associated with MG. The majority of individuals with MG have antibodies targeting acetylcholine receptors (AChR) or, less commonly, other proteins at the neuromuscular junction. Serological tests aid in confirming the autoimmune nature of the disorder.

E. Imaging Studies (CT, MRI) to Assess Thymus:

• Thymus Evaluation: As the thymus is often implicated in MG, imaging studies such as computed tomography (CT) or magnetic resonance imaging (MRI) may be employed to assess the size and condition of the thymus gland. Thymic abnormalities, including thymomas or thymic hyperplasia, may be identified.

Additional Considerations:

• Edrophonium Test: An edrophonium (Tensilon) test may sometimes be conducted. Edrophonium, a short-acting acetylcholinesterase inhibitor, is administered, and the patient is observed for a temporary improvement in muscle strength. While this test is less commonly used today, it was historically a part of the diagnostic repertoire.

Multidisciplinary Approach:

• Collaboration among Specialists: Diagnosis and management of MG often involve collaboration between neurologists, neuromuscular specialists, and other healthcare professionals. An interdisciplinary approach ensures a comprehensive understanding of the patient's condition and tailored intervention strategies.

CLASSIFICATION AND STAGING FOR INFORMED MANAGEMENT

Myasthenia Gravis (MG), a nuanced neuromuscular disorder, exhibits a spectrum of manifestations, necessitating a systematic classification based on muscle involvement and staging to guide appropriate interventions. Here are the classification and staging systems:

A. Classification Based on Muscle Involvement:

1. Ocular Myasthenia Gravis (OMG):

• Presentation: Limited to the eye muscles.

• Common Symptoms: Ptosis (drooping eyelids), diplopia (double vision).

• Prognosis: Often associated with a more favorable outcome compared to generalized MG.

2. Generalized Myasthenia Gravis:

• Presentation: Involvement of muscles beyond the eyes.

• Common Symptoms: Weakness in facial muscles,

difficulty swallowing, proximal muscle weakness.

• Subcategories:

• Early-Onset Generalized MG: Onset before age 50.

• Late-Onset Generalized MG: Onset at age 50 or older.

3. Juvenile Myasthenia Gravis:

• Presentation: Occurs in individuals under the age of 18.

• Clinical Characteristics: It resembles generalized MG but has unique considerations for pediatric care.

B. Staging (Mild, Moderate, Severe):

1. Mild MG:

• Symptoms: Generally limited to specific muscle groups, often ocular muscles.

• Impact on Daily Activities: Mild interference with daily functioning.

• Fatigue: Symptoms worsen with activity but do not significantly impede activities of daily living (ADLs).

• Management: Often managed with medications, lifestyle adjustments, and periodic follow-ups.

2. Moderate MG:

• Symptoms: Extends to involve multiple muscle groups, including facial and limb muscles.

• Impact on Daily Activities: Moderate interference with ADLs, occasional need for adjustments.

• Fatigue: Noticeable fatigue with sustained activity, requiring strategic planning of tasks.

• Management: Medications, physical therapy, and more frequent medical monitoring may be necessary.

3. Severe MG:

• Symptoms: Widespread muscle involvement, affecting multiple muscle groups.

• Impact on Daily Activities: Significant interference with ADLs, the potential need for assistance.

• Fatigue: Pronounced fatigue, even with minimal activity.

• Management: Intensive medical intervention, possibly including immunosuppressive therapy, thymectomy, and close monitoring due to the risk of respiratory complications.

4. Myasthenic Crisis:

• Emergency Situation: Represents the most severe form, characterized by respiratory failure.

• Presentation: Severe weakness of respiratory muscles, necessitating urgent medical attention.

• Management: Admission to an intensive care unit for respiratory support, intravenous immunoglobulin (IVIG), plasma exchange, and other interventions.

TREATMENT STRATEGIES

The management of Myasthenia Gravis (MG) involves a multifaceted approach, encompassing medications, surgical interventions, symptomatic treatment, and vigilant ongoing management. Here's the treatment modalities for MG:

A. Medications:

1. Acetylcholinesterase Inhibitors:

Mechanism of Action: Enhance the availability of acetylcholine at the neuromuscular junction, temporarily alleviating muscle weakness.

Common Medications: Pyridostigmine (Mestinon), neostigmine.

Usage: Often used for mild to moderate MG symptoms.

Considerations: Individualized dosing based on symptom severity and response.

2. Immunosuppressive Drugs:

Purpose: Modulate the immune system to reduce the production of antibodies attacking the neuromuscular junction.

Common Medications: Prednisone, azathioprine, mycophenolate mofetil, cyclosporine.

Usage: Particularly beneficial for individuals with moderate to severe MG or those with inadequate response to other therapies.

Considerations: Close monitoring for potential side effects, with dosage adjustments as needed.

B. Thymectomy:

Rationale: Surgical removal of the thymus gland is often recommended for individuals with thymoma or generalized MG.

Benefits: This may lead to symptom improvement and reduced reliance on medications.

Timing: Considered in early-stage MG or when thymic abnormalities are present.

Considerations: Thorough evaluation of potential benefits and risks with the healthcare team.

C. Symptomatic Treatment and Rehabilitation:

Physical Therapy: Targeted exercises to address muscle weakness, improve coordination, and enhance overall bodily function.

Speech Therapy: Beneficial for individuals with MG-related speech and swallowing difficulties.

Assistive Devices: Depending on muscle involvement, devices such as braces, walkers, or mobility aids may be recommended.

Nutritional Support: Ensuring adequate nutrition, especially in cases of difficulty swallowing.

D. Ongoing Management and Monitoring:

Regular Follow-ups: Periodic assessments with healthcare professionals to monitor symptom progression and treatment efficacy.

Medication Adjustments: Fine-tuning medication dosages based on symptom severity and potential side effects.

Immunosuppressive Monitoring: Regular blood tests to monitor blood cell counts, liver function, and other parameters for individuals on immunosuppressive drugs.

Respiratory Monitoring: Vigilant monitoring of respiratory function, especially in severe cases, to detect early signs of respiratory compromise.

Individualized Care Plans: Tailoring management strategies to each individual's evolving needs and responses.

PROGNOSIS IN MYASTHENIA GRAVIS

Understanding the prognosis of Myasthenia Gravis (MG) is a complex endeavor, given its variable and often unpredictable course. A comprehensive examination of the factors influencing prognosis provides valuable insights into the trajectory of this neuromuscular disorder:

A. Variable Course of the Disease:

1. Fluctuating Symptoms:

• Dynamic Nature: MG is characterized by a fluctuating course, marked by periods of exacerbation and remission. Symptoms may vary in intensity and can be influenced by factors such as stress, illness, or medication adjustments.

• Unpredictability: The variable nature of MG makes it challenging to predict an individual's long-term course, and the disease's experience can differ significantly among patients.

2. Ocular vs. Generalized MG:

• Ocular MG: In some cases, individuals with ocular MG

may experience a more favorable prognosis compared to those with generalized MG. Visual symptoms like ptosis and diplopia may remain isolated or progress more slowly.

3. Thymus Involvement:

• Thymectomy Impact: The presence of thymic abnormalities, such as thymomas or thymic hyperplasia, can influence prognosis. Thymectomy, especially in early-stage MG, may lead to symptom improvement and, in some cases, long-term remission.

B. Factors Influencing Prognosis:

1. Age of Onset:

• Early Onset: MG that manifests at a younger age, particularly in childhood or adolescence, may have a different clinical course compared to late-onset MG. Juvenile MG, for instance, may exhibit unique considerations and responses to treatment.

2. General Health and Lifestyle Factors:

• Overall Health: Individuals with MG who maintain good overall health, including cardiovascular fitness and respiratory function, may have a more favorable prognosis.

• Lifestyle Choices: Factors such as a balanced diet, regular exercise, and stress management can positively contribute to overall well-being, potentially influencing the course of MG.

3. Treatment Response:

• Medication Efficacy: The response to medications, including acetylcholinesterase inhibitors and immunosuppressive drugs, plays a crucial role in prognosis. Individuals who respond well to treatment and achieve stable symptom control may experience better long-term outcomes.

• Thymectomy Outcome: For those undergoing thymectomy, the success of the procedure in terms of symptom improvement and long-term remission contributes to prognosis.

4. Presence of Comorbidities:

• Impact of Other Conditions: The presence of additional health conditions or comorbidities can complicate the management of MG and influence prognosis. Collaborative management addressing multiple health aspects is essential.

5. Respiratory Involvement:

• Respiratory Function: MG with significant respiratory muscle involvement poses a higher risk of myasthenic crisis, impacting prognosis. Vigilant monitoring and timely intervention are critical in such cases.

MYASTHENIA GRAVIS LIFESTYLE AND COPING STRATEGIES

Living with Myasthenia Gravis (MG) involves a dynamic journey that demands resilience, adaptation, and a proactive approach to well-being. Adopting a set of lifestyle and coping strategies plays a pivotal role in navigating the complexities of MG and enhancing overall quality of life:

1. Knowledge Empowerment:

• Understanding MG: Knowledge is a powerful tool. Individuals with MG benefit from acquiring a deep understanding of their condition, its symptoms, triggers, and management strategies. Education facilitates informed decision-making and empowers individuals to participate in their care actively.

2. Team-Based Healthcare:

• Collaborative Care: Building a solid healthcare team is essential. Establishing open communication with neurologists, specialists, and healthcare professionals ensures a collaborative approach to managing MG.

Regular check-ups, sharing concerns, and discussing treatment plans contribute to effective care.

3. Medication Management:

• Consistent Medication Schedule: Adhering to prescribed medication schedules, including acetylcholinesterase inhibitors and immunosuppressive drugs, is crucial. Establishing a routine and utilizing medication reminders can help maintain consistency.

4. Energy Conservation:

• Balancing Activities: Recognizing the limits imposed by MG-related fatigue is vital. Distributing tasks throughout the day, incorporating breaks, and prioritizing activities help conserve energy and prevent excessive strain on muscles.

5. Stress Management:

• Mind-Body Practices: Stress can exacerbate MG symptoms. Engaging in stress-reduction techniques such as mindfulness, meditation, and deep breathing exercises can contribute to overall well-being. Identifying and addressing sources of stress is pivotal.

6. Nutrition and Hydration:

• Balanced Diet: A nutritious diet supports overall health and muscle function. Adequate hydration is crucial, especially if swallowing difficulties are present. Consultation with a nutritionist can ensure dietary choices align with MG management.

7. Physical Activity:

• Tailored Exercise: When tailored to individual capabilities, physical activity can be beneficial. Engaging in low-impact exercises under the guidance of a physical therapist helps maintain muscle strength and flexibility.

8. Adaptive Devices and Tools:

• Assistive Aids: Depending on muscle involvement, individuals may benefit from adaptive devices such as braces, mobility aids, or speech-assistive tools. These aids enhance independence and facilitate daily activities.

9. Support Networks:

• Community Engagement: Connecting with support groups, both online and offline, provides a platform for sharing experiences and insights. Peer support fosters a sense of community and understanding.

10. Emotional Well-Being: - Psychological Support: MG can impact emotional well-being. Seeking support from mental health professionals, counselors, or psychologists helps address the emotional aspects of living with a chronic condition.

11. Planning for Flare-Ups: - Emergency Preparedness: A plan for potential MG flare-ups or myasthenic crises is crucial. This includes knowing when to seek immediate medical attention and having emergency contacts readily available.

12. Adaptive Work and Lifestyle Adjustments: - Flexible Work Arrangements: Exploring flexible work options, such as remote work or modified schedules, supports individuals in managing MG while maintaining career engagement. Advocating for workplace accommodations is essential.

CHAPTER TWO

The Role of Diet in Managing Myasthenia Gravis (MG)

Myasthenia Gravis (MG), a complex neuromuscular disorder, necessitates a multifaceted approach to management. While diet alone cannot cure MG, it supports overall well-being and addresses specific challenges associated with the condition. Here are the role of diet in managing MG:

1. Balanced Nutrition for Muscle Health:

• Protein-Rich Diet: Proteins are essential for muscle health and function. Including lean protein sources such as poultry, fish, tofu, and legumes helps maintain muscle strength.

• Omega-3 Fatty Acids: Found in fatty fish, flaxseeds, and walnuts, omega-3 fatty acids have anti-inflammatory properties that may contribute to overall muscle health.

2. Adequate Hydration:

• Swallowing Difficulties: MG can lead to challenges in swallowing. Ensuring proper hydration by sipping water throughout the day and incorporating hydrating foods, such as soups and water-rich fruits, helps address this issue.

3. Small, Frequent Meals:

• Fatigue Management: MG-related fatigue can be mitigated by consuming smaller, more frequent meals throughout the day. This approach prevents energy depletion and aids in better digestion.

4. Avoidance of Trigger Foods:

• Potential Trigger Identification: Some individuals with MG may identify specific foods that exacerbate symptoms. Keeping a food diary and noting any correlations with symptom flare-ups can help identify potential triggers.

5. Vitamin and Mineral Supplementation:

• Calcium and Vitamin D: Adequate calcium and vitamin D intake is crucial for bone health, especially if individuals are on medications that may affect bone density.

• Vitamin B12: Vitamin B12, found in meat, fish, and dairy products, supports nerve health and may be supplemented if levels are deficient.

6. Careful Medication Timing:

• Interaction Considerations: Some medications for MG, such as acetylcholinesterase inhibitors, may interact with certain foods or nutrients. Consulting with healthcare professionals ensures optimal medication absorption and effectiveness.

7. Collaboration with a Nutritionist:

• Individualized Guidance: Consulting with a nutritionist or dietitian provides personalized guidance. They can tailor dietary recommendations to the individual's specific needs, taking into account factors such as weight management and nutritional deficiencies.

8. Avoidance of Alcohol and Caffeine:

• Potential Interactions: Alcohol and caffeine may interact with MG medications or contribute to muscle fatigue. Moderation or avoidance may be recommended, especially if there is a noticeable impact on symptoms.

9. Mindful Eating:

• Stress Reduction: Mindful eating, which involves paying attention to the sensory experience of eating, can help reduce stress. Stress management is crucial for individuals with MG, as stress can exacerbate symptoms.

THE IMPORTANCE OF A BALANCED AND NUTRIENT-RICH DIET

A balanced and nutrient-rich diet is a cornerstone for optimal health and well-being. Our food choices directly impact our physical and mental functions, contributing to the prevention of diseases, the promotion of vitality, and the support of various bodily functions. Here are the importance of embracing a balanced and nutrient-rich diet:

1. Essential Nutrients for Body Functions:

• Proteins: Crucial for building and repairing tissues, supporting immune function, and serving as a source of energy.

• Carbohydrates: The primary energy source for the body, fueling brain function and supporting physical activities.

• Fats: Essential for hormone production, nutrient absorption, and maintaining cell structure.

2. Vitamins and Minerals for Vitality:

• Vitamins: Play critical roles in various physiological

processes, including immune function, vision, blood clotting, and collagen formation.

• Minerals: Essential for bone health, nerve function, fluid balance, and the formation of red blood cells.

3. Disease Prevention and Management:

• Heart Health: A diet rich in fruits, vegetables, whole grains, and lean proteins supports cardiovascular health by reducing the risk of heart disease.

• Weight Management: Nutrient-dense foods contribute to a feeling of fullness, aiding in weight management and reducing the risk of obesity-related conditions.

• Diabetes Control: Balanced nutrition helps regulate blood sugar levels, supporting individuals with diabetes in managing their condition.

4. Optimal Growth and Development:

• Childhood: Adequate nutrition is crucial for children's physical and cognitive development. Proper nutrient intake supports growth, learning, and immune function.

• Adolescence: Nutrient-rich diets are essential during adolescence to support growth spurts, hormonal changes, and the development of bone density.

5. Mental Health and Cognitive Function:

• Brain Health: Nutrients like omega-3 fatty acids, antioxidants, and vitamins support cognitive function and reduce the risk of neurodegenerative diseases.

• Mood Regulation: Balanced nutrition contributes to the regulation of neurotransmitters, influencing mood and mental well-being.

6. Immune System Support:

• Antioxidants: Found in fruits and vegetables, antioxidants strengthen the immune system by neutralizing free radicals and reducing inflammation.

• Protein: Supports the production of antibodies and immune cells, crucial for defending against infections.

7. Digestive Health:

• Fiber: A diet rich in fiber promotes healthy digestion, prevents constipation, and supports gut health by fostering a diverse microbiome.

• Hydration: Proper hydration aids in digestion, nutrient absorption, and the elimination of waste products.

8. Longevity and Quality of Life:

• Reduced Chronic Diseases: A balanced diet contributes to a lower risk of chronic diseases, potentially extending life expectancy and improving overall quality of life.

• Energy and Vitality: Nutrient-rich foods provide sustained energy, supporting an active lifestyle and promoting vitality as individuals age.

9. Individualized Dietary Needs:

• Varied Requirements: Individual nutritional needs vary based on factors such as age, sex, activity level, and health conditions. A balanced diet can be tailored to meet these unique requirements.

THE IMPORTANCE OF MAINTAINING A HEALTHY WEIGHT

Maintaining a healthy weight is a cornerstone of overall well-being, influencing physical health, mental resilience, and the prevention of various chronic diseases. Striking a balance between diet, physical activity, and lifestyle choices is essential for achieving and sustaining an optimal weight. Here are the importance of maintaining a healthy weight:

1. Cardiovascular Health:

• Heart Disease Prevention: Excess weight, especially abdominal fat, is a risk factor for heart disease. Maintaining a healthy weight contributes to lower blood pressure, improved cholesterol levels, and a reduced risk of cardiovascular issues.

2. Type 2 Diabetes Prevention and Management:

• Insulin Sensitivity: Maintaining a healthy weight supports insulin sensitivity, reducing the risk of developing type 2 diabetes. For those already living with diabetes, weight management is crucial for better blood sugar control.

3. Reduced Risk of Chronic Diseases:

• Cancer: Obesity is linked to an increased risk of certain cancers, including breast, colorectal, and pancreatic cancer. Maintaining a healthy weight lowers the likelihood of developing these conditions.

• Osteoarthritis: Excess weight places strain on joints, contributing to the development and progression of osteoarthritis. Weight management is critical to mitigating joint pain and improving mobility.

4. Respiratory Health:

• Sleep Apnea: Obesity is a significant risk factor for sleep apnea, a condition characterized by disrupted breathing during sleep. Achieving a healthy weight can alleviate symptoms and improve respiratory function.

5. Mental Health and Well-Being:

• Self-Esteem and Confidence: Maintaining a healthy weight can positively impact self-esteem and confidence, fostering a positive body image and mental well-being.

• Reduced Risk of Depression: Studies suggest that weight management may contribute to a lower risk of depression, emphasizing the intricate connection between physical and mental health.

6. Improved Fertility:

• Reproductive Health: Obesity can affect reproductive health, leading to hormonal imbalances and fertility issues. Achieving and maintaining a healthy weight supports reproductive function in both men and women.

7. Joint Health and Mobility:

• Reduced Strain: Excess weight places additional strain on joints, particularly in the knees, hips, and lower back. Maintaining a healthy weight alleviates this strain, promoting joint health and reducing the risk of injuries.

8. Longevity and Quality of Life:

• Increased Life Expectancy: Research indicates that maintaining a healthy weight is associated with increased life expectancy. A lower risk of chronic diseases contributes to a longer, healthier life.

• Enhanced Quality of Life: Individuals at a healthy weight often experience improved energy levels, physical function, and overall quality of life.

9. Metabolic Health:

• Blood Sugar Regulation: Healthy weight management supports optimal blood sugar regulation, reducing the risk of metabolic syndrome and associated complications.

• Lipid Profile: Achieving and maintaining a healthy weight contributes to a favorable lipid profile, lowering the risk of atherosclerosis and related cardiovascular issues.

10. Prevention of Childhood Obesity: - Establishing Healthy Habits: Encouraging and maintaining a healthy weight in childhood sets the foundation for lifelong habits. Preventing childhood obesity reduces the risk of associated health issues in adulthood.

11. Individualized Approach to Wellness: - Unique Considerations: Recognizing that ideal weight varies among individuals, a healthy weight is context-specific and considers factors such as body composition, genetics, and lifestyle.

NUTRITIONAL REQUIREMENTS FOR OPTIMAL MUSCLE FUNCTION

Muscles, the powerhouses of the human body, require a delicate balance of nutrients to function optimally. Proper nutrition is essential for muscle growth and sustaining strength, promoting endurance, and facilitating efficient recovery. Here's a comprehensive exploration of the nutritional requirements crucial for supporting muscle function:

1. Protein for Muscle Building and Repair:

• Amino Acids: Proteins are comprised of amino acids, the building blocks of muscle tissue. Consuming adequate high-quality protein sources, such as lean meats, poultry, fish, eggs, dairy, and plant-based proteins, is vital for muscle repair and growth.

• Timing: Distributing protein intake evenly throughout the day, including post-exercise, enhances muscle protein synthesis and aids in recovery.

2. Carbohydrates for Energy:

• Fuel for Workouts: Carbohydrates serve as the body's primary energy source. Consuming complex carbohydrates, like whole grains, fruits, and vegetables, provides sustained energy for both endurance and strength-based exercises.

• Glycogen Replenishment: Carbohydrates are crucial for replenishing glycogen stores in muscles, promoting recovery after intense physical activity.

3. Fats for Hormone Production and Energy:

• Hormone Regulation: Healthy fats, including omega-3 fatty acids and monounsaturated fats, play a role in hormone production. Hormones such as testosterone influence muscle growth and repair.

• Energy Reserves: Dietary fats serve as an energy source, especially during low to moderate-intensity activities. Including sources like avocados, nuts, and olive oil supports overall energy balance.

4. Hydration for Fluid Balance:

• Electrolyte Balance: Maintaining proper hydration is crucial for optimal muscle function. Adequate fluid intake supports electrolyte balance, preventing muscle cramps and promoting efficient nerve-muscle communication.

• Exercise Considerations: During intense physical activity, especially in hot environments, maintaining electrolyte balance through sports drinks or electrolyte-rich foods is essential.

5. Vitamins and Minerals for Muscle Health:

• Calcium and Vitamin D: Essential for bone health, calcium and vitamin D play a role in muscle contractions.

Including dairy products, leafy greens, and exposure to sunlight supports these requirements.

• Iron: Adequate iron intake is crucial for oxygen transport to muscles. Iron-rich foods like lean meats, beans, and fortified cereals contribute to overall muscle health.

6. Antioxidants for Recovery:

• Combatting Oxidative Stress: Intense exercise can lead to oxidative stress and inflammation in muscles. Consuming antioxidants from fruits, vegetables, and nuts helps mitigate this stress and supports muscle recovery.

7. Branched-Chain Amino Acids (BCAAs):

• Muscle Preservation: BCAAs, including leucine, isoleucine, and valine, are essential amino acids with a role in muscle protein synthesis. Including BCAAs in the diet, either through food sources or supplements, can support muscle preservation and growth.

8. Caffeine for Endurance and Performance:

• Enhanced Endurance: Caffeine in coffee and tea has been shown to improve endurance and performance during endurance-based activities. It may also reduce the perception of effort during exercise.

9. Meal Timing for Muscle Protein Synthesis:

• Post-Exercise Nutrition: Consuming a balanced meal or snack containing protein and carbohydrates after exercise enhances muscle protein synthesis and replenishes glycogen stores. This is crucial for recovery and adaptation to training.

10. Individualized Nutrition Plans: - Unique

Requirements: Nutritional needs vary among individuals based on factors such as age, gender, activity level, and specific fitness goals. Tailoring nutrition plans to individual requirements is critical for optimal muscle function.

SPECIAL CONSIDERATIONS FOR INDIVIDUALS WITH SWALLOWING DIFFICULTIES

Swallowing difficulties, or dysphagia, can present unique challenges in maintaining proper nutrition and hydration. Individuals facing this condition require special considerations to ensure their dietary needs and overall well-being are safeguarded. Here are the critical considerations for those with swallowing difficulties:

1. Texture-Modified Diets:

• Soft and Pureed Diets: Individuals with dysphagia may benefit from texture-modified diets, such as soft or pureed foods. These diets facilitate easier swallowing and reduce the risk of aspiration.

• Consistency Adjustments: Healthcare professionals, including speech therapists and dietitians, can guide individuals in selecting foods that match their specific swallowing abilities.

2. Hydration Strategies:

• Thickened Liquids: For those with difficulty swallowing thin liquids, thickened liquids can be easier to manage. Adjusting the consistency of liquids to nectar-thick or honey-thick may help prevent aspiration.

• Water Intake Management: Ensuring adequate hydration is crucial. If thin liquids are challenging, incorporating hydrating foods with high water content, such as fruits and soups, can contribute to overall fluid intake.

3. Nutrient-Dense Foods:

• Calorie and Protein Density: Selecting nutrient-dense foods becomes essential to meet calorie and protein needs, mainly when the volume of food intake is restricted.

• Fortified Foods: Including fortified foods and nutritional supplements, under healthcare professionals' guidance, can help address potential nutrient deficiencies.

4. Mealtime Strategies:

• Small, Frequent Meals: Breaking meals into smaller, more frequent portions can make swallowing more manageable and reduce fatigue associated with eating.

• Slow and Mindful Eating: Encouraging a slow and mindful approach to eating allows individuals to focus on each bite, promoting safe swallowing and enhancing the overall dining experience.

5. Adaptable Food Preparation:

• Blending and Pureeing: Utilizing blenders and food processors to modify the texture of foods can open up a broader range of options for those with swallowing difficulties.

• Creative Cooking Techniques: Exploring innovative cooking techniques, such as mashing or slow cooking, can enhance the palatability and ease of swallowing for certain foods.

6. Assistive Devices and Tools:

• Adaptive Utensils: Specially designed utensils and plates with partitions can assist individuals in managing food and preventing spillage.

• Straws and Sippy Cups: Using straws or sippy cups can offer alternatives for safely consuming liquids.

7. Positioning During Meals:

• Optimal Seating: Proper seating and positioning during meals can promote safe swallowing. Individuals may benefit from sitting upright, with proper head and neck support.

• Posture Adjustments: Experimenting with different postures, such as tucking the chin, can help facilitate safer swallowing.

8. Collaboration with Healthcare Professionals:

• Speech Therapists: Working closely with speech therapists is essential for evaluating swallowing function, providing tailored exercises, and recommending appropriate texture-modified diets.

• Dietitians: Registered dietitians can create personalized nutrition plans, ensuring individuals with dysphagia receive adequate nutrients while accommodating their specific swallowing abilities.

9. Education and Communication: - Communication with Caregivers: Informing caregivers and family members about the individual's specific dietary needs and preferences fosters a supportive environment. - Educational Resources: Utilizing educational resources and support groups can empower individuals and their caregivers with valuable information and practical tips.

10. Regular Monitoring and Adjustments: - Dynamic Nature of Dysphagia: Dysphagia may evolve over time, necessitating regular reassessment and adjustments to the individual's diet and mealtime strategies. - Open Communication: Encouraging open communication between individuals, caregivers, and healthcare professionals ensures that any changes or challenges are addressed promptly.

RECOMMENDED NUTRIENTS FOR HOLISTIC HEALTH

Ensuring a well-rounded and nutrient-rich diet supports overall health, promotes overall health, and prevents nutritional deficiencies. Several vital nutrients play integral roles in various physiological functions, contributing to both physical and mental well-being. Here are the recommended nutrients, each with its unique benefits:

A. Antioxidants (Vitamins C and E):

• Role: Antioxidants, including vitamins C and E, play a crucial role in neutralizing free radicals unstable molecules that can damage cells and contribute to aging and disease.

• Sources: Citrus fruits, berries, leafy greens, nuts, seeds, and vegetable oils are rich sources of these antioxidants.

• Benefits: Supporting immune function, promoting skin health, and contributing to cardiovascular health are among the benefits of adequate antioxidant intake.

B. Omega-3 Fatty Acids:

• Role: Omega-3 fatty acids, particularly EPA

(eicosapentaenoic acid) and DHA (docosahexaenoic acid), are essential for brain health, cardiovascular function, and reducing inflammation.

• Sources: Fatty fish (salmon, mackerel, sardines), flaxseeds, chia seeds, and walnuts are excellent sources of omega-3 fatty acids.

• Benefits: Supporting cognitive function, reducing the risk of heart disease, and alleviating inflammatory conditions are among the benefits associated with omega-3 fatty acids.

C. Protein for Muscle Support:

• Role: Proteins are vital for building and repairing tissues, supporting immune function, and serving as a source of energy.

• Sources: Lean meats, poultry, fish, eggs, dairy products, legumes, and plant-based proteins such as tofu and tempeh are excellent protein sources.

• Benefits: Maintaining muscle mass, supporting immune health, and facilitating the synthesis of enzymes and hormones are vital benefits of adequate protein intake.

D. Vitamin D for Bone Health:

• Role: Vitamin D is crucial for the absorption of calcium and phosphorus, promoting bone health and overall immune function.

• Sources: Sun exposure, fatty fish (salmon, mackerel), fortified dairy products, and egg yolks are natural sources of vitamin D.

• Benefits: Preventing bone diseases such as osteoporosis, supporting immune function, and contributing to overall musculoskeletal health are vital benefits associated with vitamin D.

E. Calcium for Muscle Function:

• Role: Calcium is essential for bone health, muscle contraction, blood clotting, and nerve function.

• Sources: Dairy products, leafy greens (kale, broccoli), fortified plant-based milk, and certain types of fish (sardines, salmon) are rich in calcium.

• Benefits: Maintaining solid bones, supporting muscle function, and preventing osteoporosis are among the benefits associated with adequate calcium intake.

Recommendations for a Balanced Diet:

• Variety: Consuming a variety of nutrient-dense foods ensures a broad spectrum of essential nutrients.

• Whole Foods: Prioritizing entire foods over processed foods maximizes the intake of vitamins, minerals, and other beneficial compounds.

• Moderation: Balancing nutrient intake and avoiding excessive consumption of specific nutrients is essential for overall health.

Individualized Considerations:

• Age and Life Stage: Nutrient needs vary across different life stages, from childhood to older adulthood.

• Health Conditions: Individuals with specific health conditions or dietary restrictions may require personalized nutrition plans.

• Consultation with Healthcare Professionals: Seeking guidance from healthcare professionals, including nutritionists and dietitians, ensures that dietary choices align with individual health goals and requirements.

FOODS TO INCLUDE

Crafting a balanced and wholesome diet involves selecting a variety of nutrient-dense foods that provide essential vitamins, minerals, and other beneficial compounds. The following categories of foods form the pillars of a nourishing diet, contributing to overall health and vitality:

A. Lean Proteins (Chicken, Fish, Tofu):

• Role: Lean proteins are rich in essential amino acids, supporting muscle health, immune function, and overall tissue repair.

• Sources: Chicken, fish (salmon, tuna), tofu, tempeh, and legumes (beans, lentils) are excellent sources of lean proteins.

• Benefits: Promoting satiety, maintaining muscle mass, and supporting metabolic function are vital benefits associated with incorporating lean proteins into the diet.

B. Whole Grains and Complex Carbohydrates:

• Role: Whole grains and complex carbohydrates are primary sources of energy, providing sustained fuel for the body and supporting digestive health.

• Sources: Quinoa, brown rice, oats, whole wheat bread,

and sweet potatoes are examples of whole grains and complex carbohydrates.

• Benefits: Stable energy levels, improved digestion, and a rich supply of fiber and nutrients are among the benefits associated with including whole grains in the diet.

C. Colorful Fruits and Vegetables:

• Role: Colorful fruits and vegetables are rich in vitamins, minerals, antioxidants, and fiber, contributing to overall health and disease prevention.

• Sources: Berries, citrus fruits, leafy greens, bell peppers, carrots, and broccoli are vibrant examples of fruits and vegetables.

• Benefits: Supporting immune function, promoting skin health, and reducing the risk of chronic diseases are key benefits associated with a colorful array of fruits and vegetables.

D. Dairy or Dairy Alternatives for Calcium:

• Role: Dairy products and fortified dairy alternatives are essential for obtaining calcium, which is crucial for bone health, muscle function, and nerve transmission.

• Sources: Milk, yogurt, cheese, and fortified plant-based milk (soy, almond, oat) are examples of calcium-rich foods.

• Benefits: Maintaining solid bones, supporting muscle function, and preventing osteoporosis are critical benefits associated with adequate calcium intake.

Guidelines for a Balanced Diet:

• Variety: Including a diverse range of foods ensures a broad spectrum of nutrients and prevents dietary monotony.

• Portion Control: Moderation in portion sizes helps maintain a healthy balance of calorie intake and supports weight management.

• Hydration: Water is essential for overall health. Incorporating hydrating foods like fruits and vegetables contributes to overall fluid intake.

Individualized Considerations:

• Dietary Preferences: Individuals may tailor their food choices based on dietary preferences, including vegetarian, vegan, or gluten-free options.

• Health Conditions: Certain health conditions may require adjustments to the types and amounts of specific foods consumed.

• Lifestyle Factors: Consideration of lifestyle factors, such as physical activity levels and stress management, can influence dietary choices.

FOODS TO AVOID OR LIMIT

While constructing a balanced and nourishing diet, it's equally important to be mindful of foods that can contribute to health risks when consumed in excess. The following categories highlight foods that are best approached with moderation to promote overall well-being:

A. Processed and High-Sodium Foods:

• Concerns: Processed foods often contain high levels of sodium, which can contribute to elevated blood pressure and increase the risk of cardiovascular issues.

• Examples: Packaged snacks, canned soups, instant noodles, and processed meats are familiar sources of excessive sodium.

• Guidelines: Opting for fresh, whole foods and reading labels to monitor sodium content can help reduce the intake of processed and high-sodium foods.

B. Foods High in Saturated Fats:

• Concerns: Diets high in saturated fats can lead to elevated cholesterol levels, increasing the risk of heart disease and other cardiovascular conditions.

• Examples: Fatty cuts of red meat, full-fat dairy products, butter, and certain tropical oils are sources of saturated fats.

• Guidelines: Choosing leaner protein sources, incorporating plant-based fats (such as avocados and nuts), and opting for low-fat dairy products can help moderate saturated fat intake.

C. Sugary Snacks and Beverages:

• Concerns: Excessive consumption of sugary snacks and beverages is linked to weight gain, insulin resistance, and an increased risk of metabolic disorders and dental issues.

• Examples: Candy, sugary cereals, sweetened beverages, and pastries are familiar sources of added sugars.

• Guidelines: Prioritizing whole fruits for sweetness, choosing water or unsweetened beverages, and being mindful of added sugars in processed foods contribute to a healthier approach to sugar consumption.

Additional Considerations:

• Trans Fats: Foods containing trans fats, often found in partially hydrogenated oils, should be avoided. Trans fats can raise harmful cholesterol levels and increase the risk of heart disease.

• Highly Processed Snacks: Snack items like chips, cookies, and sure crackers often contain a combination of unhealthy fats, added sugars, and high levels of sodium.

Guiding Principles for Healthy Eating:

• Moderation: Enjoying foods high in sodium, saturated fats, or added sugars in moderation can be part of a balanced diet.

• Whole Foods Focus: Prioritizing whole, minimally processed foods ensures a nutrient-rich intake and minimizes exposure to added unhealthy ingredients.

• Mindful Eating: Paying attention to portion sizes, savoring the flavors of whole foods, and cultivating mindful eating habits contribute to a healthier relationship with food.

HYDRATION

Hydration is a cornerstone of overall health, influencing various bodily functions and contributing to well-being. Understanding the importance of staying hydrated and making mindful choices about beverages are crucial aspects of maintaining optimal health.

A. Importance of Staying Hydrated:

• 1. Cellular Function: Water is essential for the proper functioning of cells, facilitating nutrient transport, and supporting biochemical reactions. Adequate hydration ensures cells operate efficiently.

• 2. Temperature Regulation: Sweating, a natural cooling mechanism, helps regulate body temperature. Proper hydration is vital for maintaining this process, preventing overheating, and supporting thermal equilibrium.

• 3. Cognitive Function: Dehydration can impair cognitive function, affecting concentration, alertness, and short-term memory. Staying hydrated promotes mental clarity and overall cognitive performance.

• 4. Physical Performance: Athletes and individuals engaging in physical activities benefit from optimal hydration. Fluid balance enhances endurance, strength, and overall exercise performance.

• 5. Detoxification: Adequate water intake supports the

body's natural detoxification processes by flushing out waste products through urine, helping maintain kidney function.

B. Choosing Appropriate Beverages:

• 1. Water: Pure and calorie-free water is the optimal choice for hydration. It's readily available, supports all bodily functions, and is essential for overall well-being.

• 2. Herbal Teas: Unsweetened herbal teas provide hydration along with potential health benefits. Options like chamomile or peppermint can be soothing and refreshing.

• 3. Infused Water: Adding natural flavors to water with fruits, herbs, or vegetables can enhance taste, encouraging increased water intake.

• 4. Electrolyte Drinks: In intense physical activity situations, electrolyte drinks can help replenish electrolytes lost through sweat. However, they should be consumed in moderation, as many commercial varieties contain added sugars.

• 5. Coconut Water: A natural source of electrolytes, coconut water is a hydrating option with a mild taste. It contains potassium, magnesium, and other essential minerals.

• 6. Milk: A combination of water, electrolytes, and nutrients, milk provides hydration while offering calcium and protein. Opt for low-fat or plant-based alternatives for variety.

• 7. Limiting Sugary and Caffeinated Beverages: Sugary drinks and caffeinated beverages can contribute to dehydration if consumed in excess. While coffee and tea can contribute to overall fluid intake, moderation is key.

Guidelines for Optimal Hydration:

• 1. Listen to Thirst: Paying attention to the body's signals for thirst is a simple yet effective way to maintain proper hydration levels.

• 2. Daily Water Intake: While individual needs vary, a standard guideline is the "8x8 rule" — consuming eight 8-ounce glasses of water per day. However, factors like age, activity level, and climate influence hydration requirements.

• 3. Preemptive Hydration: Ensuring adequate hydration before engaging in physical activity or spending time in a hot environment is essential for preventing dehydration.

MONITORING AND ADAPTING THE DIET

Monitoring and adapting the diet is a dynamic process essential for promoting overall well-being, especially for individuals managing specific health conditions, symptoms, or changes in medications. Regular nutritional assessments and adjustments based on evolving circumstances play a pivotal role in optimizing dietary habits.

A. Regular Nutritional Assessments:

• 1. Periodic Check-Ins: Regular nutritional assessments conducted by healthcare professionals or registered dietitians provide a snapshot of an individual's nutritional status. These assessments may include reviewing dietary habits, nutrient intake, and potential deficiencies.

• 2. Body Composition Analysis: Tools like body mass index (BMI), waist-to-hip ratio, and body fat percentage measurements offer insights into body composition, helping tailor nutritional recommendations.

• 3. Blood Tests: Monitoring blood markers, such as cholesterol levels, blood glucose, and nutrient levels (vitamins, minerals), aids in identifying nutritional deficiencies or imbalances.

• 4. Dietary Records: Keeping detailed records of daily food intake allows individuals and healthcare professionals to analyze dietary patterns, identify trends, and make informed adjustments.

B. Adjustments Based on Changes in Symptoms or Medications:

• 1. Symptom Management: Individuals experiencing changes in symptoms related to their health condition should collaborate with healthcare professionals to adapt their diet accordingly. For example, adjusting fiber intake for gastrointestinal symptoms or modifying carbohydrate intake for blood sugar management.

• 2. Medication Interactions: Changes in medication regimens may impact nutrient absorption or metabolism. Collaboration with healthcare providers ensures that dietary adjustments align with medication requirements and potential side effects.

• 3. Allergies and Sensitivities: Developing allergies or sensitivities to certain foods may necessitate modifications to the diet. Identifying trigger foods and finding suitable alternatives is crucial for preventing adverse reactions.

• 4. Lifestyle Changes: Life events, such as pregnancy, aging, or changes in physical activity levels, require dietary adaptations. Nutrient needs vary during different life stages, and adjusting the diet to meet these changing requirements is essential.

• 5. Weight Management: Individuals working towards weight management goals may need to adjust their dietary approach based on progress and evolving health needs. This may involve modifying calorie intake, nutrient distribution, or meal timing.

Guiding Principles for Effective Adaptations:

• Open Communication: Regular communication with healthcare professionals, including dietitians, ensures that dietary adaptations align with overall health goals and medical guidance.

• Gradual Changes: Making incremental adjustments to the diet allows for better adaptation and helps individuals sustain long-term dietary habits.

• Individualized Plans: Recognizing each individual's unique needs and preferences is crucial for creating personalized dietary plans. There is no one-size-fits-all approach, and adaptations should consider the individual's lifestyle, cultural factors, and taste preferences.

Individualized Considerations:

• Chronic Conditions: Individuals managing chronic conditions, such as diabetes, cardiovascular disease, or gastrointestinal disorders, may require ongoing dietary adaptations to optimize symptom management and overall health.

• Age and Life Stage: Dietary needs change with age, and adapting the diet to meet the requirements of different life stages is vital for maintaining optimal health.

SAMPLE MEAL PLAN

Creating a well-rounded and varied meal plan is crucial for providing essential nutrients, sustaining energy levels, and promoting overall health. The following sample meal plan for seven days incorporates a diverse range of foods to offer a balanced and nourishing approach:

Day 1:

Breakfast:

• Scrambled eggs with spinach and tomatoes

• Whole-grain toast

• Fresh orange slices

Lunch:

• Grilled chicken salad with mixed greens, cherry tomatoes, cucumber, and a vinaigrette dressing

• Quinoa on the side

Snack:

• Greek yogurt with a handful of mixed berries

Dinner:

• Baked salmon with lemon and herbs

- Steamed asparagus

- Sweet potato wedges

Day 2:

Breakfast:

- Overnight oats with almond milk, chia seeds, sliced bananas, and a drizzle of honey

Lunch:

- Whole-grain wrap with turkey, avocado, lettuce, and tomato

- Carrot sticks on the side

Snack:

- Hummus with cucumber and bell pepper slices

Dinner:

- Lentil and vegetable stir-fry with brown rice

Day 3:

Breakfast:

- Smoothie bowl with mixed berries, banana, spinach, Greek yogurt, and a sprinkle of granola

Lunch:

- Quinoa and black bean stuffed bell peppers

- Mixed green salad with balsamic vinaigrette

Snack:

- Handful of almonds and an apple

Dinner:

- Grilled cod with mango salsa

- Steamed broccoli

• Quinoa on the side

Day 4:

Breakfast:

• Whole-grain toast with smashed avocado and poached eggs

• Sliced strawberries

Lunch:

• Chickpea and spinach curry

• Brown rice

Snack:

• Cottage cheese with pineapple chunks

Dinner:

• Seared tofu with vegetable medley (broccoli, bell peppers, carrots)

• Quinoa on the side

Day 5:

Breakfast:

• Greek yogurt parfait with layers of granola, mixed berries, and a drizzle of honey

Lunch:

• Turkey and vegetable stir-fry with quinoa

Snack:

• Edamame and carrot noodle stir-fry

Dinner:

• Roasted vegetable and chickpea wrap with tahini dressing

Day 6:

Breakfast:

• Whole-grain pancakes with fresh berries and a dollop of Greek yogurt

• Orange juice

Lunch:

• Quinoa salad with mixed vegetables (bell peppers, cherry tomatoes, cucumber) and feta cheese

• Grilled chicken breast on top

Snack:

• Sliced pear with almond butter

Dinner:

• Shrimp and broccoli skewers

• Brown rice

Day 7:

Breakfast:

• Avocado and walnut quinoa bowl with a sprinkle of cinnamon

• Green tea

Lunch:

• Caprese salad with tomatoes, mozzarella, and basil

• Whole-grain baguette

Snack:

• Mixed berry smoothie with spinach and chia seeds

Dinner:

• Baked salmon with dill and asparagus

- Roasted sweet potato wedges

- Roasted sweet potato wedges

SAMPLE SHOPPING LIST

Building a well-balanced and nutritious pantry starts with thoughtful grocery shopping. A well-planned shopping list ensures you have the ingredients needed for diverse and satisfying meals. Here is the sample shopping list organized by food categories:

Fresh Produce:

• Leafy greens (spinach, kale, arugula)

• Colorful vegetables (bell peppers, tomatoes, carrots, cucumbers)

• Fresh fruits (berries, apples, oranges, bananas, mangoes)

Proteins:

• Lean meats (chicken breast, turkey, lean ground beef)

• Fatty fish (salmon, cod)

• Plant-based proteins (tofu, tempeh, legumes - beans, lentils)

• Eggs

Whole Grains:

• Quinoa

• Brown rice

- Whole-grain pasta
- Oats
- Whole-grain bread or wraps

Dairy and Alternatives:

- Greek yogurt
- Low-fat or plant-based milk (almond, soy, oat)
- Feta or mozzarella cheese
- Cottage cheese

Healthy Fats:

- Avocados
- Nuts (almonds, walnuts)
- Seeds (chia seeds, flaxseeds)
- Olive oil

Herbs and Spices:

- Basil
- Cilantro
- Mint
- Garlic
- Turmeric
- Cumin
- Paprika
- Black pepper

Canned and Jarred Goods:

- Canned beans (black beans, chickpeas)
- Diced tomatoes

- Tomato sauce

- Hummus

- Nut butter (almond, peanut)

- Olives

Frozen Foods:

- Mixed berries

- Broccoli florets

- Mixed Vegetables

- Frozen shrimp or fish fillets

Bakery and Snacks:

- Whole-grain crackers

- Baked tortilla chips

- Granola

- Dark chocolate

Beverages:

- Water

- Herbal teas

- Green tea

Condiments and Sauces:

- Balsamic vinaigrette

- Olive oil-based dressing

- Soy sauce

- Mustard

- Salsa

- Tahini

Miscellaneous:

• Honey

• Whole-grain pancake mix

• Whole-grain tortillas

Considerations:

• Check for sales or discounts to optimize your budget.

• Purchase fresh produce in quantities that can be consumed before expiration.

• Consider buying in bulk for non-perishable items to reduce packaging waste.

Adaptations:

• Adjust quantities based on the number of people in your household and your meal-planning preferences.

• Tailor the list to accommodate specific dietary needs or preferences (e.g., gluten-free, vegetarian).

CHAPTER THREE

Colorful Fruits And Vegetables Recipes

Beet and Goat Cheese Salad with Walnuts

Meal Description:

Indulge in a delightful combination of earthy beets, creamy goat cheese, and crunchy walnuts with this vibrant and refreshing Beet and Goat Cheese Salad. This salad is visually appealing and packed with a medley of flavors and textures that will satisfy your taste buds.

Ingredients:

For the Salad:

• Four medium-sized beets, roasted, peeled, and sliced

• 4 cups mixed salad greens (arugula, spinach, or your choice)

• 1/2 cup goat cheese, crumbled

• 1/2 cup walnuts, toasted and roughly chopped

For the Dressing:

• Three tablespoons extra-virgin olive oil

• Two tablespoons of balsamic vinegar

• One teaspoon of Dijon mustard

• One teaspoon honey

• Salt and black pepper to taste

Optional Additions:

• Sliced red onions

• Fresh herbs (such as parsley or dill)

Instructions:

1. Prepare the Beets:

• Preheat the oven to 400°F (200°C).

• Wrap each beet individually in foil and roast in the oven for about 45-60 minutes or until they can be easily pierced with a fork.

• Once cooled, peel the beets and slice them into rounds or wedges.

2. Toast the Walnuts:

• In a dry skillet over medium heat, toast the walnuts for 3-5 minutes, stirring frequently, until they become fragrant. Be careful not to burn them. Set aside to cool.

3. Make the Dressing:

• Whisk together the olive oil, balsamic vinegar, Dijon mustard, honey, salt, and black pepper in a small bowl until well combined.

4. Assemble the Salad:

• Arrange the mixed salad greens on a serving platter or individual plates.

• Place the roasted beet slices on top of the greens.

• Sprinkle crumbled goat cheese and toasted walnuts over the beets.

5. Drizzle with Dressing:

• Drizzle the balsamic vinaigrette dressing over the salad.

6. Garnish and Serve:

• Optionally, add sliced red onions and fresh herbs for extra flavor and freshness.

• Serve the Beet and Goat Cheese Salad immediately, enjoying the combination of flavors and textures.

Nutrition Information (per serving):

• Calories: 300 calories

• Protein: 8g

• Carbohydrates: 20g

• Fat: 25g

• Fiber: 5g

RATATOUILLE WITH HERBED QUINOA

Meal Description:

Immerse yourself in Ratatouille's rich and comforting flavors paired with light and fragrant Herbed Quinoa. This classic French vegetable stew, accompanied by a bed of quinoa infused with fresh herbs, creates a harmonious and satisfying dish that celebrates the abundance of seasonal vegetables.

Ingredients:

For the Ratatouille:

- One eggplant, diced
- One zucchini, diced
- One yellow squash, diced
- One red bell pepper, diced
- One yellow bell pepper, diced
- One onion, finely chopped
- Three cloves garlic, minced
- One can (14 oz) diced tomatoes, undrained
- Two tablespoons of tomato paste
- One teaspoon of dried thyme

- One teaspoon of dried rosemary
- One teaspoon dried oregano
- Salt and black pepper to taste
- Two tablespoons olive oil

For the Herbed Quinoa:

- 1 cup quinoa, rinsed and drained
- 2 cups vegetable broth or water
- One tablespoon olive oil
- One tablespoon of fresh parsley chopped
- One tablespoon of fresh basil, chopped
- Salt and black pepper to taste

Optional Garnish:

- Fresh basil or parsley for garnish
- Grated Parmesan cheese

Instructions:

1. Prepare the Ratatouille:

- Heat olive oil over medium heat in a large pot or Dutch oven.

- Add chopped onions and minced garlic, and sauté until softened.

- Add diced eggplant, zucchini, yellow squash, red bell pepper, and yellow bell pepper. Cook for 5-7 minutes, stirring occasionally.

2. Add Tomatoes and Herbs:

- Stir in diced tomatoes, tomato paste, dried thyme, rosemary, oregano, salt, and black pepper.

• Bring the mixture to a simmer, then reduce heat to low, cover, and let it cook for 20-25 minutes or until the vegetables are tender.

3. Prepare the Herbed Quinoa:

• In a separate saucepan, combine quinoa and vegetable broth or water.

• Bring to a boil, then reduce heat to low, cover, and simmer for 15-20 minutes or until quinoa is cooked and liquid is absorbed.

• Mix the quinoa with a fork and stir in olive oil, parsley, basil, salt, and black pepper.

4. Serve:

• Spoon a generous portion of Ratatouille over a serving of Herbed Quinoa.

• Garnish with fresh basil or parsley and, if desired, sprinkle with grated Parmesan cheese.

Nutrition Information (per serving):

• Calories: 350 calories

• Protein: 10g

• Carbohydrates: 60g

• Fat: 12g

• Fiber: 10g

MANGO AVOCADO SALSA WITH BAKED TORTILLA CHIPS

Snack Description:

Delight your taste buds with the refreshing and vibrant flavors of Mango Avocado Salsa paired with crispy Baked Tortilla Chips. This colorful and wholesome snack perfectly balances sweet and savory, providing a burst of tropical goodness in every bite.

Ingredients:

For the Mango Avocado Salsa:

• Two ripe mangos, peeled, pitted, and diced

• One ripe avocado, peeled, pitted, and diced

• 1/2 red onion, finely chopped

• One jalapeño, seeded and finely chopped

• 1/4 cup fresh cilantro, chopped

• Juice of 2 limes

• Salt and black pepper to taste

For the Baked Tortilla Chips:

• 6 whole-grain tortillas

- Olive oil cooking spray

- One teaspoon of chili powder

- 1/2 teaspoon ground cumin

- Salt to taste

Instructions:

For the Mango Avocado Salsa:

1. Combine diced mangos, diced avocado, chopped red onion, chopped jalapeño, and chopped cilantro in a large bowl.

2. Squeeze the juice of two limes over the mixture.

3. Season with salt and black pepper to taste.

4. Gently toss the ingredients together until well combined.

5. Allow the salsa to chill in the refrigerator for at least 30 minutes to let the flavors meld.

For the Baked Tortilla Chips:

1. Preheat the oven to 375°F (190°C).

2. Stack the tortillas and cut them into triangles, like tortilla chips.

3. Place the tortilla triangles on a baking sheet in a single layer.

4. Lightly coat the tortillas with olive oil cooking spray.

5. Mix chili powder, ground cumin, and salt in a small bowl. Sprinkle this mixture over the tortilla triangles.

6. Bake in the preheated oven for 8-10 minutes or until the chips are golden and crispy.

Serve:

1. Arrange the baked tortilla chips around the edge of a serving platter.

2. Spoon the Mango Avocado Salsa into the center of the platter.

3. Garnish with additional cilantro if desired.

4. Serve immediately and enjoy this delightful Mango Avocado Salsa with Baked Tortilla Chips.

Nutrition Information (per serving):

• Calories: 150 calories

• Protein: 2g

• Carbohydrates: 25g

• Fat: 7g

• Fiber: 4g

WATERMELON AND FETA SALAD

Salad Description:

Experience the perfect blend of sweet and savory with this refreshing Watermelon and Feta Salad. Juicy watermelon, creamy feta cheese, and fresh mint combine to create a light and delightful salad that's both hydrating and flavorful.

Ingredients:

For the Salad:

• 4 cups cubed seedless watermelon

• 1 cup crumbled feta cheese

• 1/2 red onion, thinly sliced

• 1/4 cup fresh mint leaves, torn

• 1/4 cup black olives, pitted and sliced (optional)

• 1/4 cup balsamic glaze or reduction

For the Dressing:

• Two tablespoons extra-virgin olive oil

• One tablespoon of balsamic vinegar

• Salt and black pepper to taste

Instructions:

1. Prepare the Watermelon:

• Cut the watermelon into bite-sized cubes, discarding the seeds.

2. Assemble the Salad:

• In a large salad bowl, combine the cubed watermelon, crumbled feta cheese, thinly sliced red onion, torn mint leaves, and sliced black olives (if using).

3. Make the Dressing:

• Whisk together olive oil, balsamic vinegar, salt, and black pepper in a small bowl to create the dressing.

4. Dress the Salad:

• Drizzle the dressing over the watermelon and feta mixture.

5. Toss Gently:

• Gently toss the salad ingredients to ensure an even coating of the dressing.

6. Drizzle with Balsamic Glaze:

• Drizzle balsamic glaze or reduction over the salad for an extra burst of flavor.

7. Serve:

• Transfer the Watermelon and Feta Salad to a serving platter or individual plates.

8. Garnish and Enjoy:

• Garnish with additional fresh mint leaves.

• Serve immediately and enjoy the refreshing combination of sweet watermelon, salty feta, and the brightness of mint.

Nutrition Information (per serving):

- Calories: 200 calories
- Protein: 5g
- Carbohydrates: 25g
- Fat: 10g
- Fiber: 2g

ROASTED VEGETABLE AND CHICKPEA WRAP

Wrap Description:

Enjoy a burst of Mediterranean flavors with this delicious and nutritious Roasted Vegetable and Chickpea Wrap. This wrap is a satisfying and wholesome meal, packed with roasted vegetables, protein-rich chickpeas, and a zesty tahini dressing.

Ingredients:

For the Roasted Vegetables and Chickpeas:

• 1 cup cherry tomatoes, halved

• One red bell pepper, sliced

• One zucchini, sliced

• One small red onion, sliced

• One can (15 oz) chickpeas, drained and rinsed

• Two tablespoons olive oil

• One teaspoon of ground cumin

• One teaspoon of smoked paprika

• Salt and black pepper to taste

For the Tahini Dressing:

• Three tablespoons tahini

• Two tablespoons of lemon juice

• One clove of garlic, minced

• One teaspoon of honey or maple syrup

• Two tablespoons water (more if needed)

• Salt and black pepper to taste

For the Wrap:

• Whole-grain wraps or tortillas

• Fresh spinach or mixed greens

• Feta cheese, crumbled (optional)

• Fresh herbs (parsley, cilantro), chopped

Instructions:

1. Roast the Vegetables and Chickpeas:

• Preheat the oven to 400°F (200°C).

• In a large bowl, combine cherry tomatoes, sliced red bell pepper, sliced zucchini, sliced red onion, and chickpeas.

• Drizzle with olive oil and sprinkle with ground cumin, smoked paprika, salt, and black pepper. Toss to coat.

• Spread the mixture on a baking sheet in a single layer.

• Roast in the preheated oven for 20-25 minutes or until the vegetables are tender and slightly caramelized.

2. Prepare the Tahini Dressing:

• Whisk together tahini, lemon juice, minced garlic, honey or maple syrup, water, salt, and black pepper in a small bowl until smooth. Adjust the consistency with more water if needed.

3. Assemble the Wrap:

• Warm the whole-grain wraps or tortillas according to package instructions.

• Spread a generous spoonful of the tahini dressing on each wrap.

• Layer with fresh spinach or mixed greens.

4. Add Roasted Vegetables and Chickpeas:

• Spoon the roasted vegetable and chickpea mixture onto the wraps.

5. Garnish and Serve:

• Optional: Crumble feta cheese over the top.

• Sprinkle with chopped fresh herbs.

• Fold the sides of the wrap and roll it up.

6. Serve Immediately:

• Slice the wrap in half diagonally and serve immediately.

Nutrition Information (per serving):

• Calories: 400 calories

• Protein: 12g

• Carbohydrates: 45g

• Fat: 20g

• Fiber: 10g

SPINACH AND FRUIT SALAD WITH CITRUS VINAIGRETTE

Salad Description:

Indulge in a refreshing and vibrant Spinach and Fruit Salad with Citrus Vinaigrette. This delightful salad combines nutrient-rich spinach with a medley of fresh fruits and a zesty citrus dressing, creating a perfect balance of flavors and textures.

Ingredients:

For the Salad:

- 4 cups fresh baby spinach leaves, washed and dried
- 1 cup strawberries, hulled and sliced
- 1 cup blueberries
- 1 cup mandarin orange segments
- 1/2 cup sliced almonds, toasted
- 1/4 cup crumbled feta cheese (optional)

For the Citrus Vinaigrette:

- Three tablespoons extra-virgin olive oil
- Two tablespoons of fresh orange juice
- One tablespoon of fresh lemon juice
- One teaspoon of Dijon mustard
- One teaspoon of honey or maple syrup
- Salt and black pepper to taste

Instructions:

1. Prepare the Citrus Vinaigrette:

- In a small bowl, whisk together extra-virgin olive oil, fresh orange juice, fresh lemon juice, Dijon mustard, honey or maple syrup, salt, and black pepper until well combined.

2. Toast the Almonds:

- In a dry skillet over medium heat, toast the sliced almonds for 3-5 minutes, stirring frequently, until they become golden and fragrant. Be careful not to burn them. Set aside to cool.

3. Assemble the Salad:

- Combine fresh baby spinach leaves, sliced strawberries, blueberries, mandarin orange segments, and toasted sliced almonds in a large salad bowl.

4. Add Optional Feta:

- Optional: Sprinkle crumbled feta cheese over the salad for an extra burst of flavor.

5. Drizzle with Citrus Vinaigrette:

- Drizzle the prepared citrus vinaigrette over the salad.

6. Toss Gently:

• Gently toss the salad to ensure an even coating of the dressing.

7. Serve:

• Divide the Spinach and Fruit Salad onto individual plates.

8. Garnish and Enjoy:

• Garnish with additional sliced almonds and, if desired, more crumbled feta cheese.

• Serve immediately and enjoy the refreshing combination of spinach, fresh fruits, and citrusy vinaigrette.

Nutrition Information (per serving):

• Calories: 250 calories

• Protein: 5g

• Carbohydrates: 20g

• Fat: 18g

• Fiber: 5g

SWEET POTATO AND KALE HASH

Meal Description:

Start your day right with the hearty and nutritious Sweet Potato and Kale Hash. Packed with the goodness of sweet potatoes, Kale, and savory spices, this flavorful hash makes for a satisfying breakfast or a wholesome side dish.

Ingredients:

• Two medium sweet potatoes, peeled and diced

• 2 cups kale, stems removed and chopped

• One red onion, diced

• Two cloves garlic, minced

• One teaspoon of smoked paprika

• One teaspoon of ground cumin

• 1/2 teaspoon chili powder

• Salt and black pepper to taste

• Two tablespoons olive oil

• Four eggs (optional for serving)

• Fresh parsley or cilantro for garnish

Instructions:

1. Prepare Sweet Potatoes:

• Peel and dice the sweet potatoes into small, bite-sized cubes.

2. Sauté Vegetables:

• In a large skillet, heat olive oil over medium heat.

• Add diced red onion and minced garlic. Sauté until softened.

3. Add Sweet Potatoes:

• Add the diced sweet potatoes to the skillet. Cook for about 10-15 minutes or until the sweet potatoes are tender, stirring occasionally.

4. Season the Hash:

• Sprinkle smoked paprika, ground cumin, chili powder, salt, and black pepper over the sweet potatoes. Mix well to coat evenly.

5. Add Kale:

• Add chopped Kale to the skillet. Cook for an additional 3-5 minutes or until the Kale is wilted and tender.

6. Optional Eggs:

• Create small wells in the hash and crack eggs into each well if you'd like to include eggs. Cover the skillet and cook until the eggs are cooked to your liking.

7. Garnish:

• Garnish the Sweet Potato and Kale Hash with fresh parsley or cilantro.

8. Serve:

• Divide the hash onto plates or serve it family-style.

Nutrition Information (per serving, without eggs):

- Calories: 200 calories
- Protein: 4g
- Carbohydrates: 30g
- Fat: 8g
- Fiber: 5g

CAPRESE SALAD WITH TOMATOES, MOZZARELLA, AND BASIL

Salad Description:

Savor the simplicity of a classic Caprese Salad, where the vibrant colors and flavors of ripe tomatoes, fresh mozzarella, and fragrant basil come together to create a light and refreshing dish. This Italian salad is perfect for showcasing the beauty of summer produce.

Ingredients:

For the Salad:

• Four large ripe tomatoes, sliced

• 1 pound fresh mozzarella cheese, sliced

• Fresh basil leaves

• Extra-virgin olive oil

• Balsamic glaze or reduction (optional)

• Salt and black pepper to taste

Instructions:

1. Arrange Tomatoes and Mozzarella:

• On a serving platter, alternate slices of ripe tomatoes and fresh mozzarella.

2. Add Basil Leaves:

• Tuck fresh basil leaves between the tomato and mozzarella slices.

3. Drizzle with Olive Oil:

• Drizzle extra-virgin olive oil over the tomato and mozzarella slices.

4. Season with Salt and Pepper:

• Sprinkle salt and black pepper to taste over the salad.

5. Optional Balsamic Glaze:

• Optional: Drizzle balsamic glaze or reduction over the Caprese Salad for extra sweetness and tanginess.

6. Serve:

• Serve the Caprese Salad immediately, allowing the flavors to meld.

7. Garnish (Optional):

• Garnish with additional fresh basil leaves.

Nutrition Information (per serving):

• Calories: 250 calories

• Protein: 15g

• Carbohydrates: 5g

• Fat: 20g

• Fiber: 2g

MIXED BERRY SMOOTHIE BOWL

Smoothie Bowl Description:

Start your day with a burst of energy and a symphony of flavors with this vibrant Mixed Berry Smoothie Bowl. Packed with antioxidants, vitamins, and natural sweetness, this bowl is delicious and a nourishing way to kickstart your morning.

Ingredients:

For the Smoothie Base:

• 1 cup mixed berries (strawberries, blueberries, raspberries, blackberries)

• One ripe banana, frozen

• 1/2 cup Greek yogurt

• 1/2 cup almond milk (or any milk of your choice)

• One tablespoon of honey or maple syrup (optional for added sweetness)

Toppings:

• Granola

• Sliced strawberries

• Blueberries

- Chia seeds

- Shredded coconut

- Fresh mint leaves

Instructions:

1. Prepare the Smoothie Base:

- Combine mixed berries, frozen banana, Greek yogurt, and almond milk in a blender.

- Blend until smooth and creamy. Add honey or maple syrup if you prefer a sweeter taste.

2. Pour into a Bowl:

- Pour the smoothie into a bowl, ensuring a smooth and even surface.

3. Add Toppings:

- Sprinkle granola generously over the smoothie base.

4. Arrange Fresh Berries:

- Decorate the bowl with sliced strawberries and blueberries.

5. Enhance with Chia Seeds and Coconut:

- Sprinkle chia seeds and shredded coconut for added texture and nutritional benefits.

6. Garnish with Fresh Mint:

- Garnish the Mixed Berry Smoothie Bowl with fresh mint leaves for a burst of freshness.

7. Serve:

- Serve the smoothie bowl immediately and enjoy the combination of creamy smoothie base and crunchy toppings.

Nutrition Information:

- Calories: 300 calories
- Protein: 10g
- Carbohydrates: 50g
- Fat: 8g
- Fiber: 8g

RAINBOW VEGGIE STIR-FRY WITH BROWN RICE

Stir-Fry Description:

Indulge in a burst of colors and flavors with this Rainbow Veggie Stir-Fry with Brown Rice. Packed with an array of fresh vegetables and served over wholesome brown rice, this dish is a nutritious and delicious way to enjoy the goodness of plant-based ingredients.

Ingredients:

For the Stir-Fry:

- 1 cup broccoli florets
- One bell pepper (red or yellow), sliced
- One carrot, julienned
- 1 cup snap peas, ends trimmed
- 1 cup shredded purple cabbage
- 1 cup sliced mushrooms
- One tablespoon of vegetable oil
- Two cloves garlic, minced
- One tablespoon ginger, grated

- Two tablespoons of low-sodium soy sauce

- One tablespoon of hoisin sauce

- One tablespoon of rice vinegar

- One teaspoon of sesame oil

- Sesame seeds for garnish (optional)

For the Brown Rice:

- 1 cup brown rice

- 2 cups water

- 1/2 teaspoon salt

Instructions:

For the Brown Rice:

1. In a medium saucepan, combine brown rice, water, and salt.

2. Bring to a boil, then reduce heat to low, cover, and simmer for 45-50 minutes or until rice is tender and water is absorbed.

3. Fluff the rice with a fork.

For the Stir-Fry:

1. In a wok or large skillet, heat vegetable oil over medium-high heat.

2. Add minced garlic and grated ginger. Sauté for 1-2 minutes until fragrant.

3. Add broccoli, bell pepper, carrot, snap peas, purple cabbage, and mushrooms to the wok. Stir-fry for 5-7 minutes or until the vegetables are tender-crisp.

4. Mix soy sauce, hoisin sauce, rice vinegar, and sesame oil in a small bowl.

5. Pour the sauce over the vegetables and toss to coat evenly. Cook for an additional 2-3 minutes.

6. Adjust seasoning to taste and remove from heat.

Assembly:

1. Spoon the Rainbow Veggie Stir-Fry over a serving of brown rice.

2. Garnish with sesame seeds if desired.

3. Serve immediately and enjoy this colorful and wholesome meal.

Nutrition Information:

• Calories: 350 calories

• Protein: 10g

• Carbohydrates: 70g

• Fat: 8g

• Fiber: 10g

CHAPTER FOUR

Lean Proteins Recipes

Grilled Lemon Herb Chicken Breast with Quinoa

Meal Description:

Savor the delightful combination of zesty lemon and aromatic herbs with our Grilled Lemon Herb Chicken Breast served over a bed of nutritious quinoa. This light and flavorful dish is perfect for a wholesome, low-calorie meal that doesn't compromise on taste.

Ingredients:

For the Chicken:

- Four boneless, skinless chicken breasts

- Two tablespoons olive oil

- One tablespoon of fresh lemon juice

- Two teaspoons of dried oregano

- One teaspoon of dried thyme

- One teaspoon of garlic powder

- Salt and black pepper to taste

For the Quinoa:

- 1 cup quinoa, rinsed and drained

- 2 cups water or chicken broth

- One tablespoon olive oil

- Salt to taste

For Garnish:

- Fresh parsley, chopped

- Lemon wedges

Instructions:

1. Marinate the Chicken:

• Mix olive oil, lemon juice, dried oregano, dried thyme, garlic powder, salt, and black pepper in a bowl.

• Place chicken breasts in a resealable plastic bag and pour the marinade over them.

• Seal the bag, ensuring the chicken is well coated. Marinate in the refrigerator for at least 30 minutes.

2. Prepare the Quinoa:

• In a medium saucepan, combine quinoa and water or chicken broth.

• Bring to a boil, then reduce heat to low, cover, and simmer for 15-20 minutes until quinoa is cooked and water is absorbed.

• Fluff the quinoa with a fork, stir in olive oil, and season with salt to taste.

3. Grill the Chicken:

• Preheat the grill to medium-high heat.

• Remove chicken from the marinade and grill for 6-8 minutes per side or until fully cooked and grill marks appear.

• Discard the marinade.

4. Assemble the Dish:

• Place a generous scoop of quinoa on each plate.

• Top with grilled lemon herb chicken breasts.

• Garnish with chopped fresh parsley and lemon wedges.

5. Serve and Enjoy:

• Serve immediately, and enjoy the burst of flavors from the grilled lemon herb chicken and nutty quinoa.

Nutrition Information (per serving):

• Calories: 230 calories

• Protein: 25g

• Carbohydrates: 15g

• Fat: 8g

• Fiber: 2g

BAKED SALMON WITH DILL AND ASPARAGUS

Meal Description:

Experience a burst of freshness with our Baked Salmon with Dill and Asparagus. This simple yet elegant dish combines succulent salmon fillets seasoned with aromatic dill, perfectly complemented by tender roasted asparagus. Enjoy a delightful and nutritious meal that's quick and easy to prepare.

Ingredients:

For the Salmon:

- Four salmon fillets

- Two tablespoons olive oil

- 2 tablespoons fresh dill, chopped

- One tablespoon of Dijon mustard

- Two cloves garlic, minced

- Salt and black pepper to taste

- Lemon wedges for serving

For the Asparagus:

- One bunch of fresh asparagus, trimmed

- One tablespoon olive oil

- Salt and black pepper to taste

Instructions:

1. Preheat the Oven:

- Preheat your Oven to 400°F (200°C).

2. Prepare the Salmon Marinade:

- Whisk together olive oil, chopped fresh dill, Dijon mustard, minced garlic, salt, and black pepper in a small bowl.

3. Marinate the Salmon:

- Place salmon fillets on a baking sheet lined with parchment paper.

- Brush the salmon fillets with the dill marinade, ensuring they are well coated.

4. Prepare the Asparagus:

- On the same baking sheet, arrange the trimmed asparagus spears.

- Drizzle with olive oil and sprinkle with salt and black pepper. Toss to coat evenly.

5. Bake in the Oven:

- Bake in the preheated Oven for 12-15 minutes or until the salmon is cooked and flakes easily with a fork.

6. Serve:

- Carefully transfer the salmon fillets and asparagus to serving plates.

- Squeeze fresh lemon juice over the salmon fillets.

• Garnish with additional fresh dill if desired.

7. Enjoy:

• Serve immediately and relish in the delicious combination of baked salmon with dill and perfectly roasted asparagus.

Nutrition Information (per serving):

• Calories: 300 calories

• Protein: 30g

• Carbohydrates: 5g

• Fat: 18g

• Fiber: 2g

TURKEY AND VEGETABLE STIR-FRY

Meal Description:

Experience a quick and nutritious delight with our Turkey and Vegetable Stir-Fry. Lean ground turkey meets a colorful array of crisp vegetables in a savory stir-fry sauce, creating a well-balanced dish that's both satisfying and full of flavor.

Ingredients:

For the Stir-Fry:

- 1 lb lean ground turkey
- Two tablespoons of vegetable oil
- One red bell pepper, thinly sliced
- 1 yellow bell pepper, thinly sliced
- 1 medium carrot, julienned
- 1 cup broccoli florets
- 1 cup snap peas, ends trimmed
- Three green onions, chopped
- Three cloves garlic, minced

• One tablespoon of fresh ginger, grated

• Sesame seeds for garnish (optional)

For the Stir-Fry Sauce:

• 1/4 cup low-sodium soy sauce

• Two tablespoons of oyster sauce

• One tablespoon of hoisin sauce

• One tablespoon of rice vinegar

• One teaspoon of sesame oil

• 1 teaspoon cornstarch

Instructions:

1. Prepare the Stir-Fry Sauce:

• Whisk together soy sauce, oyster sauce, hoisin sauce, rice vinegar, sesame oil, and cornstarch in a small bowl. Set aside.

2. Cook the Ground Turkey:

• Heat one tablespoon of vegetable oil over medium-high heat in a large wok or skillet.

• Add the ground turkey and cook, breaking it apart with a spoon, until browned and cooked through. Remove excess fat.

3. Sauté Vegetables:

• Push the cooked turkey to one side of the wok. Add the remaining one tablespoon of vegetable oil to the empty side.

• Add garlic and ginger, and sauté for 30 seconds.

• Add bell peppers, carrots, broccoli, and snap peas. Stir-fry for 3-4 minutes or until vegetables are crisp-tender.

4. Combine and Sauce:

• Mix the sautéed vegetables with the cooked turkey in the wok.

• Pour the stir-fry sauce over the turkey and vegetables. Stir well to coat evenly.

• Cook for an additional 2-3 minutes until the sauce thickens.

5. Garnish and Serve:

• Sprinkle chopped green onions and sesame seeds over the stir-fry.

• Serve the turkey and vegetable stir-fry over rice or noodles.

Nutrition Information (per serving):

• Calories: 350 calories

• Protein: 30g

• Carbohydrates: 20g

• Fat: 18g

• Fiber: 5g

LENTIL AND SPINACH SOUP WITH LEAN GROUND TURKEY

Meal Description:

Warm up with a hearty and nutritious Lentil and Spinach Soup featuring lean ground turkey. Packed with protein, fiber, and a medley of wholesome ingredients, this comforting soup is delicious and a perfect option for a well-balanced meal.

Ingredients:

For the Soup:

- 1 lb lean ground turkey
- 1 cup dried green or brown lentils, rinsed and drained
- One onion, finely chopped
- Two carrots diced
- Two celery stalks, diced
- Three cloves garlic, minced
- One teaspoon cumin

- 1 teaspoon paprika

- 1/2 teaspoon coriander

- 6 cups low-sodium chicken or vegetable broth

- One can (14 oz) diced tomatoes, undrained

- 4 cups fresh Spinach, roughly chopped

- Salt and black pepper to taste

- Olive oil for cooking

For Garnish:

- Fresh parsley, chopped

- Lemon wedges

Instructions:

1. Brown the Turkey:

- Heat a drizzle of olive oil over medium-high heat in a large pot.

- Add lean ground turkey, cook until browned, and break it apart with a spoon. Remove any excess fat.

2. Sauté Aromatics:

- Add chopped onion, carrots, and celery to the pot. Sauté until vegetables are softened, about 5 minutes.

- Add minced garlic, cumin, paprika, and coriander. Cook for an additional 1-2 minutes until fragrant.

3. Add Lentils and Broth:

- Stir in rinsed lentils, diced tomatoes (with juice), and chicken or vegetable broth.

- Bring the soup to a boil, then reduce heat to low, cover, and simmer for 25-30 minutes or until lentils are tender.

4. Incorporate Spinach:

• Add chopped Spinach to the soup and stir until wilted.

• Season with salt and black pepper to taste.

5. Serve:

• Ladle the soup into bowls.

• Garnish with fresh parsley and serve with lemon wedges on the side.

Nutrition Information (per serving):

• Calories: 300 calories

• Protein: 25g

• Carbohydrates: 30g

• Fat: 10g

• Fiber: 10g

SHRIMP AND BROCCOLI SKEWERS

Meal Description:

Elevate your dining experience with these delightful Shrimp and Broccoli Skewers. Succulent shrimp paired with tender broccoli, grilled to perfection and infused with a zesty marinade, create a light and flavorful dish that's perfect for a quick and healthy meal.

Ingredients:

For the Marinade:

- Two tablespoons olive oil
- Two tablespoons of soy sauce
- One tablespoon honey
- One tablespoon of fresh lemon juice
- Two cloves garlic, minced
- One teaspoon of grated ginger
- 1/2 teaspoon red pepper flakes (optional)
- Salt and black pepper to taste

For the Skewers:

- 1 lb large shrimp, peeled and deveined

- 2 cups broccoli florets

- Wooden or metal skewers (if using wooden skewers, soak them in water for 30 minutes before threading)

For Garnish:

- Fresh cilantro or parsley, chopped

- Sesame seeds (optional)

- Lemon wedges

Instructions:

1. Prepare the Marinade:

- Whisk together olive oil, soy sauce, honey, lemon juice, minced garlic, grated ginger, red pepper flakes (if using), salt, and black pepper.

2. Marinate the Shrimp:

- Place the shrimp in a resealable plastic bag or shallow dish.

- Pour half of the marinade over the shrimp, ensuring they are well coated. Reserve the remaining marinade for basting.

3. Blanch the Broccoli:

- Bring a pot of water to a boil. Add the broccoli florets and blanch for 2 minutes.

- Drain and immediately transfer the broccoli to an ice bath to stop cooking. Pat dry.

4. Assemble the Skewers:

- Preheat the grill or grill pan over medium-high heat.

- Thread shrimp and blanched broccoli alternately onto

skewers.

5. Grill the Skewers:

• Place the skewers on the preheated grill.

• Grill for 2-3 minutes on each side or until the shrimp are opaque and cooked through, basting with the reserved marinade.

6. Garnish and Serve:

• Sprinkle with chopped cilantro or parsley and sesame seeds (if using).

• Serve the shrimp and broccoli skewers with lemon wedges on the side.

Nutrition Information (per serving):

• Calories: 200 calories

• Protein: 20g

• Carbohydrates: 12g

• Fat: 8g

• Fiber: 3g

GREEK YOGURT CHICKEN SALAD

Meal Description:

Indulge in a healthier twist on the classic chicken salad with our Greek Yogurt Chicken Salad. Creamy Greek yogurt replaces traditional mayonnaise, creating a light and protein-packed dish that's bursting with Mediterranean flavors. Perfect for sandwiches, wraps, or serving on a bed of greens.

Ingredients:

For the Chicken Salad:

- 2 cups cooked chicken breasts, shredded or diced

- 1 cup Greek yogurt (plain, non-fat)

- 1 cucumber, finely diced

- 1 cup cherry tomatoes, halved

- 1/2 red onion, finely chopped

- 1/2 cup Kalamata olives, pitted and sliced

- 1/2 cup feta cheese, crumbled

- 1/4 cup fresh parsley, chopped

- Salt and black pepper to taste

For the Dressing:

- Two tablespoons olive oil
- One tablespoon of red wine vinegar
- One teaspoon of Dijon mustard
- One clove of garlic, minced
- One teaspoon dried oregano
- Salt and black pepper to taste

For Serving (Optional):

- Whole-grain bread, wraps, or salad greens

Instructions:

1. Prepare the Dressing:

- Whisk together olive oil, red wine vinegar, Dijon mustard, minced garlic, dried oregano, salt, and black pepper in a small bowl. Set aside.

2. Combine Chicken Salad Ingredients:

- Combine the shredded or diced chicken, Greek yogurt, cucumber, cherry tomatoes, red onion, Kalamata olives, feta cheese, and chopped parsley in a large mixing bowl.

3. Add the Dressing:

- Pour the prepared dressing over the chicken salad mixture.

- Gently toss until all ingredients are well coated with the dressing.

4. Season to Taste:

- Season the chicken salad with salt and black pepper to taste. Adjust the Seasoning as needed.

5. Serve:

- Refrigerate the chicken salad for at least 30 minutes to

allow the flavors to meld.

• Serve the Greek Yogurt Chicken Salad on whole-grain bread, wraps, or a bed of salad greens.

Nutrition Information (per serving, without bread or wraps):

• Calories: 250 calories

• Protein: 30g

• Carbohydrates: 10g

• Fat: 12g

• Fiber: 2g

SEARED TOFU WITH VEGETABLE MEDLEY

Meal Description:

Savor the goodness of plant-based cuisine with our Seared Tofu with Vegetable Medley. Perfectly seared tofu and a colorful array of fresh vegetables create a light, flavorful, satisfying, and nutritious dish.

Ingredients:

For the Seared Tofu:

• One block of firm tofu pressed and cut into cubes

• Two tablespoons of soy sauce

• One tablespoon of sesame oil

• One tablespoon cornstarch

• One tablespoon of vegetable oil for searing

For the Vegetable Medley:

• 1 cup broccoli florets

• One bell pepper, thinly sliced (any color)

• One carrot, julienned

• One zucchini, sliced

- 1 cup snap peas, ends trimmed

- Three green onions, sliced

- Two cloves garlic, minced

- One tablespoon ginger, grated

For the Sauce:

- Three tablespoons soy sauce

- One tablespoon of rice vinegar

- One tablespoon of maple syrup or agave nectar

- One teaspoon of sesame oil

For Garnish:

- Sesame seeds

- Fresh cilantro or parsley, chopped

Instructions:

1. Prepare the Seared Tofu:

- Combine soy sauce, sesame oil, and cornstarch in a bowl to make the marinade.

- Toss tofu cubes in the marinade, ensuring they are well coated.

- Heat vegetable oil in a skillet over medium-high heat.

- Sear tofu cubes until golden brown on all sides. Set aside.

2. Sauté Vegetables:

- In the same skillet, add a bit more oil if needed.

- Sauté garlic and ginger until fragrant.

- Add broccoli, bell pepper, carrot, zucchini, and snap peas. Stir-fry for 5-7 minutes or until vegetables are tender-crisp.

3. Make the Sauce:

• Whisk together soy sauce, rice vinegar, maple syrup or agave nectar, and sesame oil in a small bowl.

4. Combine Tofu, Vegetables, and Sauce:

• Add the seared tofu back to the skillet with the sautéed vegetables.

• Pour the sauce over the tofu and vegetables.

• Toss gently until everything is well coated in the sauce.

5. Garnish and Serve:

• Garnish with sesame seeds and chopped cilantro or parsley.

• Serve the Seared Tofu with Vegetable Medley over rice or noodles.

Nutrition Information (per serving, without rice or noodles):

• Calories: 250 calories

• Protein: 15g

• Carbohydrates: 20g

• Fat: 15g

• Fiber: 5g

WHITE BEAN AND CHICKEN CHILI

Meal Description:

Warm up with a comforting bowl of White Bean and Chicken Chili, a hearty and flavorful dish that combines tender chicken, creamy white beans, and a medley of spices. Perfect for a cozy meal that's easy to prepare and sure to satisfy your taste buds.

Ingredients:

For the Chili:

• 1 lb boneless, skinless chicken breasts, cooked and shredded

• Two tablespoons olive oil

• One large onion, diced

• Three cloves garlic, minced

• Two cans (15 oz each) of white beans (cannellini or Great Northern), drained and rinsed

• One can (4 oz) diced green chilies

• One teaspoon of ground cumin

• One teaspoon dried oregano

• 1/2 teaspoon ground coriander

- 1/2 teaspoon chili powder

- 4 cups chicken broth

- Salt and black pepper to taste

For Garnish:

- Fresh cilantro, chopped

- Sour cream or Greek yogurt

- Shredded Monterey Jack or cheddar cheese

- Sliced green onions

- Lime wedges

Instructions:

1. Cook and Shred the Chicken:

- Cook the chicken breasts by boiling or baking until fully cooked. Shred the chicken using two forks and set aside.

2. Sauté Aromatics:

- In a large pot, heat olive oil over medium heat.

- Add diced onion and sauté until softened, about 3-4 minutes.

- Add minced garlic and cook for an additional 1-2 minutes until fragrant.

3. Build the Chili:

- Add shredded chicken, white beans, diced green chilies, ground cumin, dried oregano, ground coriander, and chili powder to the pot. Stir to combine.

- Pour in chicken broth and bring the mixture to a simmer.

- Season with salt and black pepper to taste.

4. Simmer:

• Allow the chili to simmer for at least 20-30 minutes to let the flavors meld and the beans become tender.

5. Adjust Seasoning:

• Taste and adjust the Seasoning if needed. Add more salt, pepper, or chili powder according to your preference.

6. Serve:

• Ladle the White Bean and Chicken Chili into bowls.

• Garnish with chopped cilantro, a dollop of sour cream or Greek yogurt, shredded cheese, sliced green onions, and lime wedges.

Nutrition Information (per serving):

• Calories: 300 calories

• Protein: 25g

• Carbohydrates: 30g

• Fat: 10g

• Fiber: 8g

GRILLED COD WITH MANGO SALSA

Meal Description:

Elevate your seafood experience with Grilled Cod topped with a vibrant Mango Salsa. This dish combines the mild and flaky cod with the sweet and tangy flavors of fresh mango salsa, creating a light and refreshing meal that's perfect for warm days.

Ingredients:

For the Grilled Cod:

- Four cod fillets (about 6 oz each)

- Two tablespoons olive oil

- One teaspoon paprika

- One teaspoon of garlic powder

- Salt and black pepper to taste

- Fresh lemon wedges for serving

For the Mango Salsa:

- Two ripe mangos, peeled, pitted, and diced

- 1/2 red onion, finely chopped

- One red bell pepper, diced

- One jalapeño, seeded and finely chopped

• 1/4 cup fresh cilantro, chopped

• Juice of 1 lime

• Salt to taste

Instructions:

1. Prepare the Grilled Cod:

• Preheat the grill to medium-high heat.

• Mix olive oil, paprika, garlic powder, salt, and black pepper in a small bowl to create the marinade.

• Brush the cod fillets with the marinade on both sides.

2. Grill the Cod:

• Place the cod fillets on the preheated grill.

• Grill for 4-5 minutes per side or until the fish flakes easily with a fork and has an excellent grill mark.

3. Make the Mango Salsa:

• Combine diced mangos, red onion, red bell pepper, jalapeño, cilantro, lime juice, and a pinch of salt in a medium bowl. Mix well.

4. Serve:

• Place grilled cod fillets on plates.

• Spoon mango salsa generously over each fillet.

• Garnish with additional cilantro and serve with fresh lemon wedges on the side.

Nutrition Information (per serving):

• Calories: 250 calories

• Protein: 25g

• Carbohydrates: 20g

- Fat: 10g
- Fiber: 3g

QUINOA AND BLACK BEAN STUFFED BELL PEPPERS

Meal Description:

Savor a wholesome and protein-packed delight with these Quinoa and Black Bean Stuffed Bell Peppers. This vegetarian dish combines the nutty flavor of quinoa, the richness of black beans, and a medley of veggies, all stuffed into colorful bell peppers and baked to perfection.

Ingredients:

For the Stuffed Bell Peppers:

• Four large bell peppers (any color), halved and seeds removed

• 1 cup quinoa, cooked according to package instructions

• One can (15 oz) black beans, drained and rinsed

• 1 cup corn kernels (fresh or frozen)

• 1 cup cherry tomatoes, diced

• 1/2 red onion, finely chopped

• Two cloves garlic, minced

- One teaspoon of ground cumin

- One teaspoon of chili powder

- Salt and black pepper to taste

- 1 cup shredded cheese (cheddar or Mexican blend), optional

For Garnish:

- Fresh cilantro, chopped

- Avocado slices

- Greek yogurt or sour cream

Instructions:

1. Preheat the Oven:

- Preheat the Oven to 375°F (190°C).

2. Prepare the Quinoa and Veggies:

- Cook quinoa according to package instructions.

- Combine cooked quinoa, black beans, corn, cherry tomatoes, red onion, minced garlic, ground cumin, chili powder, salt, and black pepper in a large bowl. Mix well.

3. Stuff the Bell Peppers:

- Fill each bell pepper half with the quinoa and black bean mixture.

- If desired, sprinkle shredded cheese on top of each stuffed pepper.

4. Bake:

- Place the stuffed bell peppers on a baking sheet.

- Bake in the preheated Oven for 25-30 minutes or until the peppers are tender.

5. Garnish and Serve:

• Remove from the Oven and garnish with chopped cilantro.

• Serve the Quinoa and Black Bean Stuffed Bell Peppers with avocado slices and a dollop of Greek yogurt or sour cream on the side.

Nutrition Information (per serving, without cheese):

• Calories: 300 calories

• Protein: 10g

• Carbohydrates: 55g

• Fat: 5g

• Fiber: 8g

CHAPTER FIVE

Essential Fatty Acids Recipes

Baked Salmon with Lemon and Olive Oil

Main Course Description:

Elevate your dinner with the simplicity and exquisite flavors of Baked Salmon with Lemon and Olive Oil. This dish allows the natural goodness of Salmon to shine, enhanced by the zesty brightness of lemon and the richness of olive oil. It's a quick and healthy recipe that's perfect for a weeknight dinner or a special occasion.

Ingredients:

• Four salmon fillets (about 6 oz each), skin-on or skinless

• Two lemons, thinly sliced

• Three tablespoons extra-virgin olive oil

• Salt and black pepper to taste

• Fresh dill or parsley for garnish (optional)

Instructions:

1. Preheat the Oven:

• Preheat your oven to 375°F (190°C).

2. Prepare the Salmon:

• Pat the Salmon fillets dry with paper towels.

• Season both sides of the Salmon with salt and black pepper.

3. Arrange Lemon Slices:

• Place a sheet of parchment paper on a baking sheet.

• Arrange half of the lemon slices on the parchment paper to create a bed for the Salmon.

4. Place Salmon on Lemon Bed:

• Lay the seasoned salmon fillets on top of the bed of lemon slices.

5. Drizzle with Olive Oil:

• Drizzle extra-virgin olive oil over the salmon fillets.

6. Top with More Lemon Slices:

• Place the remaining lemon slices on top of the Salmon.

7. Bake:

• Bake in the preheated oven for 15-20 minutes or until the Salmon is cooked through and flakes easily with a fork. Cooking time may vary based on the thickness of the fillets.

8. Garnish and Serve:

• Garnish with fresh dill or parsley if desired.

• Serve the Baked Salmon with Lemon and Olive Oil immediately, allowing the citrusy aroma to tantalize your senses.

Nutrition Information (per serving):

• Calories: 300 calories

• Protein: 30g

• Carbohydrates: 3g

• Fat: 20g

• Fiber: 1g

AVOCADO AND WALNUT QUINOA BOWL

Bowl Description:

Savor the wholesome goodness of an Avocado and Walnut Quinoa Bowl—a nutritious and flavorful combination of creamy avocado, crunchy walnuts, and protein-packed quinoa quinoa. This bowl is delicious and a great source of essential nutrients for a satisfying and nourishing meal.

Ingredients:

For the Quinoa:

- 1 cup quinoa, rinsed and drained

- 2 cups vegetable broth or water

- 1/2 teaspoon salt

For the Bowl:

- One ripe avocado, sliced

- 1/2 cup walnuts, toasted and chopped

- 1 cup cherry tomatoes, halved

- 1/4 cup red onion, finely chopped

- 1/4 cup feta cheese, crumbled (optional)

- Fresh cilantro or parsley for garnish

For the Dressing:

- Three tablespoons extra-virgin olive oil

- One tablespoon of balsamic vinegar

- One teaspoon of Dijon mustard

- Salt and black pepper to taste

Instructions:

1. Prepare QuinoaQuinoa:

- Combine QuinoaQuinoa, vegetable broth or water, and salt in a medium saucepan.

- Bring to a boil, then reduce heat to low, cover, and simmer for 15-20 minutes or until QuinoaQuinoa is cooked and liquid is absorbed.

- Fluff the QuinoaQuinoa with a fork and set aside.

2. Toast Walnuts:

- In a dry skillet over medium heat, toast the walnuts for 3-5 minutes, stirring frequently, until they become fragrant. Be careful not to burn them. Set aside to cool.

3. Make the Dressing:

- In a small bowl, whisk together extra-virgin olive oil, balsamic vinegar, Dijon mustard, salt, and black pepper until well combined.

4. Assemble the Bowl:

- Divide the cooked quinoa among serving bowls.

5. Arrange Toppings:

- If using, top the quinoa with sliced avocado, toasted

walnuts, cherry tomatoes, chopped red onion, and crumbled feta cheese.

6. Drizzle with Dressing:

• Drizzle the balsamic vinaigrette dressing over the bowl.

7. Garnish and Serve:

• Garnish with fresh cilantro or parsley.

• Serve the Avocado and Walnut Quinoa Bowl immediately, enjoying the mix of textures and flavors.

Nutrition Information (per serving):

• Calories: 400 calories

• Protein: 10g

• Carbohydrates: 40g

• Fat: 25g

• Fiber: 7g

FLAXSEED AND BERRY SMOOTHIE

Smoothie Description:

Kickstart your day with a nutrient-packed Flaxseed and Berry Smoothie. This delicious and energizing blend of antioxidant-rich berries, creamy yogurt, and flaxseed nutritional powerhouse will leave you feeling refreshed and ready to tackle the day.

Ingredients:

• 1 cup mixed berries (strawberries, blueberries, raspberries)

• One ripe banana

• 1/2 cup Greek yogurt

• One tablespoon of ground flaxseed

• One tablespoon of honey or maple syrup (optional for added sweetness)

• 1 cup almond milk (or any milk of your choice)

• Ice cubes (optional)

Instructions:

1. Prepare Ingredients:

• Wash and clean the berries. Peel the ripe banana.

1. Blend the Ingredients:

• In a blender, combine mixed berries, ripe banana, Greek yogurt, ground flaxseed, honey or maple syrup (if using), and almond milk.

• Optionally, add a handful of ice cubes for a colder and thicker consistency.

1. Blend Until Smooth:

• Blend the ingredients until you achieve a smooth and creamy consistency.

1. Taste and Adjust:

• Taste the smoothie and adjust sweetness if needed by adding more honey or maple syrup.

1. Serve:

• Pour the Flaxseed and Berry Smoothie into a glass.

1. Optional Garnish:

• Garnish with a few whole berries or a sprinkle of ground flaxseed.

1. Enjoy:

• Enjoy the refreshing and nutritious Flaxseed and Berry Smoothie to fuel your day.

Nutrition Information:

• Calories: 250 calories

• Protein: 10g

• Carbohydrates: 40g

• Fat: 7g

• Fiber: 8g

GRILLED MACKEREL WITH GARLIC AND HERBS

Main Course Description:

Experience the rich and savory flavors of Grilled Mackerel with Garlic and Herbs. This dish celebrates the natural taste of mackerel while infusing it with the aromatic goodness of garlic and herbs. This simple and delicious recipe is perfect for a light and flavorful seafood dinner.

Ingredients:

- Four mackerel fillets
- Four cloves garlic, minced
- Two tablespoons fresh parsley, finely chopped
- One tablespoon of fresh thyme, chopped
- One tablespoon of fresh rosemary chopped
- Zest of 1 lemon
- Juice of 1 lemon
- Three tablespoons olive oil
- Salt and black pepper to taste
- Lemon wedges for serving

Instructions:

1. Preheat the Grill:

• Preheat your grill to medium-high heat.

2. Prepare the Marinade:

• Combine minced garlic, chopped parsley, thyme, rosemary, lemon zest, lemon juice, and olive oil in a bowl. Mix well.

3. Marinate the Mackerel:

• Pat the mackerel fillets dry with paper towels.

• Brush the fillets with the prepared garlic and herb marinade, ensuring even coverage on both sides.

• Allow the mackerel to marinate for at least 15-20 minutes.

4. Season with Salt and Pepper:

• Season the marinated mackerel fillets with salt and black pepper to taste.

5. Grill the Mackerel:

• Place the mackerel fillets on the preheated grill.

• Grill for 4-5 minutes on each side or until the fish is cooked through and quickly flakes with a fork.

6. Baste with Marinade:

• While grilling, baste the fillets with the remaining garlic and herb marinade to enhance the flavors.

7. Serve:

• Transfer the grilled mackerel to a serving platter.

• Garnish with additional fresh herbs if desired.

• Serve with lemon wedges on the side.

Nutrition Information (per serving):

• Calories: 250 calories

• Protein: 20g

• Carbohydrates: 2g

• Fat: 18g

• Fiber: 1g

CHIA SEED PUDDING WITH BERRIES

Dessert or Breakfast Pudding Description:

Indulge in a delightful and nutritious treat with Chia Seed Pudding with Berries. This easy-to-make pudding is delicious and packed with the goodness of chia seeds and the vibrant flavors of fresh berries. Enjoy it as a healthy dessert or a satisfying breakfast option.

Ingredients:

For the Chia Seed Pudding:

• 1/4 cup chia seeds

• 1 cup almond milk (or any milk of your choice)

• One tablespoon of honey or maple syrup

• 1/2 teaspoon vanilla extract

For the Toppings:

• Fresh berries (strawberries, blueberries, raspberries)

• Sliced kiwi or other fruits

• Mint leaves for garnish (optional)

• Granola or nuts (optional)

Instructions:

1. Prepare the Chia Seed Pudding:

• Combine chia seeds, almond milk, honey or maple syrup, and vanilla extract in a bowl.

• Whisk the ingredients together until well combined.

• Let the mixture sit for 5 minutes, then whisk again to avoid clumping.

• Cover the bowl and refrigerate for at least 2-3 hours or overnight to allow the chia seeds to absorb the liquid and create a pudding-like consistency.

2. Assemble the Pudding:

• Once the chia seed pudding has set, give it a good stir to ensure an even texture.

3. Serve:

• Spoon the chia seed pudding into serving glasses or bowls.

4. Add Toppings:

• Top the pudding with a generous amount of fresh berries and sliced kiwi.

• Optional: Add a sprinkle of granola or nuts for added crunch.

5. Garnish:

• Garnish with mint leaves for a pop of freshness (optional).

6. Enjoy:

• Serve the Chia Seed Pudding with Berries immediately and enjoy this nutritious and delicious treat.

Nutrition Information (per serving):

- Calories: 200 calories
- Protein: 5g
- Carbohydrates: 30g
- Fat: 8g
- Fiber: 10g

WALNUT-CRUSTED TILAPIA

Main Course Description:

Elevate your dinner with the delightful combination of crunchy walnuts and tender Tilapia in this Walnut-Crusted Tilapia recipe. The nutty coating adds a flavorful twist to the mild taste of Tilapia, creating a delicious and easy-to-prepare dish.

Ingredients:

For the Walnut Crust:

- 1 cup walnuts, finely chopped

- 1/2 cup breadcrumbs (preferably whole wheat)

- One teaspoon of dried thyme

- One teaspoon paprika

- Salt and black pepper to taste

For the Tilapia:

- Four tilapia fillets

- Two tablespoons of Dijon mustard

- Two tablespoons olive oil

- Lemon wedges for serving

Instructions:

1. Preheat the Oven:

• Preheat your oven to 400°F (200°C).

2. Prepare the Walnut Crust:

• Combine finely chopped walnuts, breadcrumbs, dried thyme, paprika, salt, and black pepper in a shallow dish. Mix well to create the walnut crust.

3. Coat Tilapia with Dijon Mustard:

• Brush each tilapia fillet with Dijon mustard, ensuring an even coating on both sides.

4. Press in the Walnut Crust:

• Press the mustard-coated tilapia fillets into the walnut crust, ensuring that the crust adheres to the fish on both sides.

5. Place on Baking Sheet:

• Place the walnut-crusted tilapia fillets on a baking sheet lined with parchment paper.

6. Drizzle with Olive Oil:

• Drizzle olive oil over the top of each fillet to promote a golden and crispy crust during baking.

7. Bake:

• Bake in the preheated oven for 12-15 minutes or until the Tilapia is cooked through and the crust is golden brown.

8. Serve:

• Serve the Walnut-Crusted Tilapia hot, with lemon wedges on the side.

Nutrition Information (per serving):

- Calories: 300 calories
- Protein: 25g
- Carbohydrates: 10g
- Fat: 20g
- Fiber: 3g

ROASTED BRUSSELS SPROUTS WITH ALMONDS

Side Dish Description:

Transform Brussels sprouts into a flavorful and nutritious delight with this Roasted Brussels Sprouts with Almonds recipe. The combination of crispy Brussels sprouts and toasted almonds creates a savory and satisfying dish, making it a perfect side for any meal.

Ingredients:

• 1 pound Brussels sprouts, trimmed and halved

• 1/2 cup almonds, sliced or chopped

• Two tablespoons olive oil

• Two cloves garlic, minced

• One teaspoon of lemon zest

• Salt and black pepper to taste

Instructions:

1. Preheat the Oven:

• Preheat your oven to 400°F (200°C).

2. Prepare Brussels Sprouts:

• Trim the ends of the Brussels sprouts and cut them in half.

3. Toss with Olive Oil:

• Toss the halved Brussels sprouts in a large bowl with olive oil, minced garlic, lemon zest, salt, and black pepper until evenly coated.

4. Arrange on Baking Sheet:

• Spread the Brussels sprouts in a single layer on a baking sheet.

5. Roast in the Oven:

• Roast in the preheated oven for 20-25 minutes or until the Brussels sprouts are golden brown and crispy on the edges. Stir halfway through the roasting time for even cooking.

6. Toast Almonds:

• In the last 5 minutes of roasting, sprinkle the sliced or chopped almonds over the Brussels sprouts. This allows the almonds to toast and become golden.

7. Serve:

• Transfer the Roasted Brussels Sprouts with Almonds to a serving dish.

• Adjust the seasoning if necessary.

• Serve hot and enjoy as a delightful side dish.

Nutrition Information (per serving):

• Calories: 150 calories

- Protein: 5g
- Carbohydrates: 12g
- Fat: 10g
- Fiber: 6g

SESAME GINGER SALMON SUSHI BOWL

Bowl Description:

Enjoy the vibrant flavors of sushi in a convenient bowl format with this Sesame Ginger Salmon Sushi Bowl. Packed with fresh Salmon, crisp vegetables, and the delightful combination of sesame and ginger, this bowl is a deconstructed sushi experience that's easy to prepare at home.

Ingredients:

For the Salmon:

- 1 pound sushi-grade Salmon, cubed

- Two tablespoons of soy sauce

- One tablespoon of sesame oil

- One tablespoon of rice vinegar

- One tablespoon of honey or maple syrup

- One teaspoon of fresh ginger, grated

For the Sushi Bowl:

- 2 cups sushi rice, cooked

- One cucumber, julienned

- One carrot, julienned

- One avocado, sliced

- One nori sheet, cut into thin strips

- Sesame seeds for garnish

- Green onions, chopped, for garnish

For the Sesame Ginger Sauce:

- Two tablespoons of soy sauce

- One tablespoon of sesame oil

- One tablespoon of rice vinegar

- One teaspoon of honey or maple syrup

- One teaspoon of fresh ginger, grated

Instructions:

1. Prepare Salmon:

- Combine soy sauce, sesame oil, rice vinegar, honey or maple syrup, and grated ginger in a bowl to create a marinade.

- Add the cubed Salmon to the marinade, ensuring it's well coated. Let it marinate for at least 15-20 minutes.

2. Cook Sushi Rice:

- Cook sushi rice according to package instructions.

3. Prepare Sesame Ginger Sauce:

- Whisk together soy sauce, sesame oil, rice vinegar, honey, or maple syrup, and grated ginger in a small bowl. Set aside.

4. Assemble Sushi Bowl:

• In serving bowls, arrange a portion of cooked sushi rice.

• Top with marinated Salmon, julienned cucumber, julienned carrot, sliced avocado, and nori strips.

5. Drizzle with Sesame Ginger Sauce:

• Drizzle the Sesame Ginger Sauce over the sushi bowl.

6. Garnish:

• Garnish with sesame seeds and chopped green onions.

7. Serve:

• Serve the Sesame Ginger Salmon Sushi Bowl immediately, offering a delectable sushi experience in a bowl.

Nutrition Information (per serving):

• Calories: 400 calories

• Protein: 25g

• Carbohydrates: 45g

• Fat: 15g

• Fiber: 5g

AVOCADO AND TUNA SALAD LETTUCE WRAPS

Lettuce Wrap Description:

Savor the freshness and simplicity of Avocado and Tuna Salad Lettuce Wraps—a light and satisfying meal that combines creamy avocado, flavorful tuna, and crisp lettuce leaves. This recipe is delicious and a healthy and low-carb alternative to traditional wraps.

Ingredients:

For the Tuna Salad:

• Two cans (5 oz each) of tuna, drained

• One ripe avocado, mashed

• 1/4 cup red onion, finely diced

• 1/4 cup celery, finely chopped

• Two tablespoons mayonnaise

• One tablespoon of Dijon mustard

• Salt and black pepper to taste

• Lemon juice (optional for added freshness)

For the Lettuce Wraps:

• Large iceberg or butter lettuce leaves, washed and patted dry

Optional Toppings:

• Cherry tomatoes, halved

• Cucumber, sliced

• Radishes, thinly sliced

• Fresh cilantro or parsley, chopped

Instructions:

1. Prepare Tuna Salad:

• Combine drained tuna, mashed avocado, diced red onion, chopped celery, mayonnaise, Dijon mustard, salt, and black pepper in a bowl.

• Mix well until all ingredients are evenly combined.

• Adjust seasoning and add lemon juice if desired.

2. Assemble Lettuce Wraps:

• Place a few spoonfuls of the tuna salad mixture onto each lettuce leaf.

3. Add Optional Toppings:

• If desired, add cherry tomatoes, cucumber slices, radish slices, or fresh herbs on top of the tuna salad.

4. Fold and Serve:

• Gently fold the lettuce leaves to create a wrap, securing the filling inside.

• Arrange the Avocado and Tuna Salad Lettuce Wraps on a serving platter.

5. Serve:

• Serve immediately, and enjoy this light and refreshing

meal.

Nutrition Information (per serving, two lettuce wraps):

- Calories: 300 calories
- Protein: 25g
- Carbohydrates: 10g
- Fat: 20g
- Fiber: 5g

CHAPTER SIX

Recommended Nutrient Foods Recipes

Spinach and Berry Salad with Balsamic Vinaigrette

Salad Description:

Enjoy a burst of freshness with this vibrant Spinach and Berry Salad. Packed with nutrient-rich Spinach, juicy berries, and a tangy balsamic vinaigrette, this salad combines sweet and savory flavors.

Ingredients:

For the Salad:

- 6 cups fresh baby spinach, washed and dried
- 1 cup strawberries, hulled and sliced
- 1/2 cup blueberries
- 1/2 cup raspberries
- 1/4 cup sliced almonds, toasted
- 1/4 cup crumbled feta cheese (optional)

For the Balsamic Vinaigrette:

- Three tablespoons extra-virgin olive oil
- Two tablespoons of balsamic vinegar
- One teaspoon of Dijon mustard
- One teaspoon of honey or maple syrup
- Salt and black pepper to taste

Instructions:

1. Prepare the Salad:

- Combine the fresh baby spinach, sliced strawberries, blueberries, raspberries, and toasted sliced almonds in a large salad bowl.

2. Make the Balsamic Vinaigrette:

• In a small bowl, whisk together extra-virgin olive oil, balsamic vinegar, Dijon mustard, honey or maple syrup, salt, and black pepper until well combined.

3. Toss the Salad:

• Drizzle the balsamic vinaigrette over the salad.

4. Toss Gently:

• Gently toss the salad to ensure the dressing coats all the ingredients evenly.

5. Garnish with Feta (Optional):

• If desired, sprinkle crumbled feta cheese over the salad for an extra layer of flavor.

6. Serve:

• Serve the Spinach and Berry Salad immediately, enjoying the combination of sweet berries, crunchy almonds, and tangy vinaigrette.

Nutrition Information (per serving):

• Calories: 250 calories

• Protein: 5g

• Carbohydrates: 20g

• Fat: 18g

• Fiber: 6g

CHICKPEA AND SPINACH CURRY

Curry Description:

Indulge in the aromatic flavors of Chickpea and Spinach Curry. This hearty and wholesome dish combines chickpeas' protein-packed goodness with Spinach's vibrant taste in a rich and flavorful curry sauce. This recipe is not only delicious but also a nutritious addition to your menu.

Ingredients:

- Two cans (15 oz each) of chickpeas, drained and rinsed
- One large onion, finely chopped
- Three cloves garlic, minced
- One tablespoon ginger, grated
- One can (14 oz) diced tomatoes
- One can (14 oz) coconut milk
- One teaspoon of ground cumin
- One teaspoon of ground coriander
- One teaspoon of turmeric powder
- One teaspoon of garam masala
- 1/2 teaspoon chili powder (adjust to taste)

- 1/2 teaspoon cayenne pepper (optional, for extra heat)
- One tablespoon of vegetable oil
- Salt and black pepper to taste
- 4 cups fresh spinach leaves, washed
- Fresh cilantro, chopped, for garnish
- Cooked basmati rice or naan bread for serving

Instructions:

1. Sauté Aromatics:

- In a large pan, heat vegetable oil over medium heat. Add chopped onions and sauté until translucent.

2. Add Garlic and Ginger:

- Add minced garlic and grated ginger to the onions. Sauté for an additional 1-2 minutes until fragrant.

3. Spice it Up:

- Stir in ground cumin, coriander, turmeric powder, garam masala, chili powder, and cayenne pepper (if used). Cook the spices for 1-2 minutes to enhance their flavors.

4. Add Tomatoes:

- Pour in the diced tomatoes with their juices. Cook for 5 minutes, allowing the tomatoes to break down and create a thick sauce.

5. Introduce Chickpeas:

- Add the drained and rinsed chickpeas to the tomato sauce. Stir well to coat the chickpeas with the spices.

6. Pour in Coconut Milk:

- Pour in the coconut milk, stirring to combine. Season with salt and black pepper to taste.

7. Simmer:

• Bring the curry to a gentle simmer. Let it cook for 15-20 minutes, allowing the flavors to meld and the chickpeas to absorb the curry sauce.

8. Add Spinach:

• In the last 5 minutes of cooking, add the fresh spinach leaves. Stir until the spinach wilts into the curry.

9. Garnish and Serve:

• Garnish the Chickpea and Spinach Curry with chopped cilantro.

• Serve the curry over cooked basmati rice or with naan bread.

Nutrition Information (per serving):

• Calories: 400 calories

• Protein: 12g

• Carbohydrates: 40g

• Fat: 25g

• Fiber: 10g

BERRY AND KALE SMOOTHIE

Smoothie Description:

Start your day on a nutritious note with this refreshing Berry and Kale Smoothie. Packed with the goodness of vibrant berries and nutrient-rich kale, this smoothie is delicious and a powerhouse of vitamins and antioxidants.

Ingredients:

• 1 cup kale leaves, stems removed and chopped

• 1/2 cup strawberries, hulled

• 1/2 cup blueberries

• 1/2 cup raspberries

• One banana, peeled

• 1/2 cup Greek yogurt

• One tablespoon of chia seeds

• 1 cup almond milk (or any milk of your choice)

• Ice cubes (optional)

Instructions:

1. Prepare Ingredients:

• Wash and prepare the kale by removing the stems and

chopping the leaves.

• Hull the strawberries and peel the banana.

2. Blend Greens and Berries:

• Combine kale leaves, strawberries, blueberries, raspberries, bananas, Greek yogurt, and chia seeds in a blender.

3. Add Liquid:

• Pour in almond milk to help with blending. Add ice cubes if you desire a colder and thicker consistency.

4. Blend Until Smooth:

• Blend the ingredients until you achieve a smooth and creamy consistency.

5. Taste and Adjust:

• Taste the smoothie and adjust sweetness or thickness by adding more banana or honey if needed.

6. Serve:

• Pour the Berry and Kale Smoothie into a glass.

7. Enjoy:

• Enjoy the refreshing and nutrient-packed Berry and Kale Smoothie to kickstart your day.

Nutrition Information:

• Calories: 250 calories

• Protein: 10g

• Carbohydrates: 40g

• Fat: 8g

• Fiber: 10g

QUINOA SALAD WITH MIXED VEGETABLES

Salad Description:

Delight in the wholesome goodness of Quinoa Salad with Mixed Vegetables—a nutritious and flavorful dish that combines protein-rich quinoa with a colorful array of fresh vegetables. This salad is not only satisfying but also a great way to incorporate a variety of nutrients into your meal.

Ingredients:

For the Quinoa:

• 1 cup quinoa, rinsed

• 2 cups water or vegetable broth

• 1/2 teaspoon salt

For the Salad:

• 1 cup cherry tomatoes, halved

• One cucumber, diced

• One bell pepper (any color), diced

• 1/2 red onion, finely chopped

- 1/2 cup Kalamata olives, pitted and sliced
- 1/4 cup fresh parsley, chopped

For the Dressing:

- Three tablespoons extra-virgin olive oil
- Two tablespoons of balsamic vinegar
- One teaspoon of Dijon mustard
- One clove of garlic, minced
- Salt and black pepper to taste

Instructions:

1. Cook Quinoa:

- Combine quinoa, water or vegetable broth, and salt in a saucepan. Bring to a boil, then reduce heat to low, cover, and simmer for 15-20 minutes or until quinoa is cooked and Liquid is absorbed. Fluff with a fork and let it cool.

2. Prepare Vegetables:

- Combine cherry tomatoes, cucumber, bell pepper, chopped red onion, sliced Kalamata olives, and fresh parsley in a large salad bowl.

3. Make the Dressing:

- In a small bowl, whisk together extra-virgin olive oil, balsamic vinegar, Dijon mustard, minced garlic, salt, and black pepper until well combined.

4. Assemble the Salad:

- Add the cooked and cooled quinoa to the bowl with the mixed vegetables.

5. Drizzle with Dressing:

- Drizzle the balsamic vinaigrette dressing over the

quinoa and vegetables.

6. Toss Gently:

• Gently toss the salad until the ingredients are well combined and coated with the dressing.

7. Serve:

• Immediately serve the Quinoa Salad with Mixed Vegetables as a light and nutritious meal.

Nutrition Information (per serving):

• Calories: 300 calories

• Protein: 8g

• Carbohydrates: 40g

• Fat: 15g

• Fiber: 6g

BROCCOLI AND CASHEW STIR-FRY

Stir-Fry Description:

Indulge in the perfect blend of crisp broccoli, crunchy cashews, and savory stir-fry sauce with this delicious and nutritious Broccoli and Cashew Stir-Fry. This quick and easy recipe is a flavorful way to enjoy a variety of textures and wholesome ingredients in one delightful dish.

Ingredients:

For the Stir-Fry:

• 2 cups broccoli florets

• 1 cup snap peas, trimmed

• One red bell pepper, sliced

• One carrot, julienned

• 1 cup baby corn, halved

• 1 cup cashews, toasted

• Three green onions, sliced (white and green parts separated)

• Sesame seeds for garnish (optional)

• Cooking oil (vegetable or sesame oil)

For the Stir-Fry Sauce:

- 1/4 cup low-sodium soy sauce

- Two tablespoons of oyster sauce

- One tablespoon of hoisin sauce

- One tablespoon of rice vinegar

- One tablespoon of honey or maple syrup

- Two teaspoons cornstarch mixed with two tablespoons water (cornstarch slurry)

Instructions:

1. Toast Cashews:

- In a dry pan over medium heat, toast the cashews until they become golden brown. Set aside.

2. Prepare Stir-Fry Sauce:

- Whisk together soy sauce, oyster sauce, hoisin sauce, rice vinegar, honey or maple syrup, and the cornstarch slurry in a bowl. Set aside.

3. Stir-Fry Vegetables:

- Heat a wok or large skillet over high heat. Add a tablespoon of oil.

- Add the broccoli, snap peas, red bell pepper, julienned carrot, and baby corn. Stir-fry for 3-4 minutes until the vegetables are crisp-tender.

4. Add SauceSauce:

- Pour the prepared stir-fry sauce over the vegetables. Toss to coat evenly.

5. Incorporate Cashews:

- Add the toasted cashews and sliced green onions (white parts). Toss again to combine.

6. Finish and Garnish:

• Cook for an additional 2 minutes, allowing the sauce to thicken and coat the vegetables.

• If desired, garnish with sliced green onions (green parts) and sesame seeds.

7. Serve:

• Serve the Broccoli and Cashew Stir-Fry hot over rice or noodles.

Nutrition Information (per serving):

• Calories: 350 calories

• Protein: 10g

• Carbohydrates: 30g

• Fat: 20g

• Fiber: 6g

GREEK QUINOA BOWL WITH TOMATOES AND CUCUMBERS

Bowl Description:

Savor the fresh and vibrant flavors of the Mediterranean with this Greek Quinoa Bowl. Packed with nutritious ingredients like quinoa, cherry tomatoes, cucumbers, olives, and feta cheese, this bowl is a delightful and wholesome option for a light and satisfying meal.

Ingredients:

For the Quinoa:

- 1 cup quinoa, rinsed

- 2 cups water or vegetable broth

- 1/2 teaspoon salt

For the Bowl:

- 1 cup cherry tomatoes, halved

- One cucumber, diced

- 1/2 red onion, thinly sliced

- 1/2 cup Kalamata olives, pitted and sliced
- 1/2 cup crumbled feta cheese
- Fresh oregano or basil for garnish

For the Greek Dressing:

- Three tablespoons extra-virgin olive oil
- Two tablespoons of red wine vinegar
- One teaspoon of Dijon mustard
- One clove of garlic, minced
- One teaspoon dried oregano
- Salt and black pepper to taste

Instructions:

1. Cook Quinoa:

• Combine quinoa, water or vegetable broth, and salt in a saucepan. Bring to a boil, then reduce heat to low, cover, and simmer for 15-20 minutes or until quinoa is cooked and Liquid is absorbed. Fluff with a fork and let it cool.

2. Prepare Greek Dressing:

• Whisk together extra-virgin olive oil, red wine vinegar, Dijon mustard, minced garlic, dried oregano, salt, and black pepper in a small bowl to create the Greek dressing.

3. Assemble the Bowl:

• Combine the cooked and cooled quinoa with cherry tomatoes, diced cucumber, thinly sliced red onion, sliced Kalamata olives, and crumbled feta cheese in a large bowl.

4. Drizzle with Dressing:

• Drizzle the Greek dressing over the quinoa and

vegetables.

5. Toss Gently:

• Gently toss the ingredients until well coated with the dressing.

6. Garnish:

• Garnish the Greek Quinoa Bowl with fresh oregano or basil.

7. Serve:

• Serve the Greek Quinoa Bowl as a light and refreshing meal.

Nutrition Information (per serving):

• Calories: 400 calories

• Protein: 10g

• Carbohydrates: 40g

• Fat: 25g

• Fiber: 6g

BERRY ALMOND OVERNIGHT OATS

Overnight Oats Description:

Kickstart your morning with the delicious and nutritious combination of berries and almonds in these Berry Almond Overnight Oats. With the convenience of preparing them the night before, you'll wake up to a ready-to-eat breakfast that's packed with fiber, antioxidants, and energy-boosting goodness.

Ingredients:

• 1/2 cup rolled oats

• 1/2 cup almond milk (or any milk of your choice)

• 1/4 cup Greek yogurt

• 1/2 cup mixed berries (strawberries, blueberries, raspberries)

• One tablespoon of almond butter

• One tablespoon of chia seeds

• One tablespoon of honey or maple syrup (optional for sweetness)

• Sliced almonds for topping

• Fresh mint leaves for garnish (optional)

Instructions:

1. Assemble the Base:

• Combine rolled oats, almond milk, Greek yogurt, and chia seeds in a mason jar or airtight container.

2. Add Berries:

• Layer the mixed berries on top of the oat mixture.

3. Swirl in Almond Butter:

• Drizzle almond butter over the berries in a swirling pattern.

4. Sweeten if Desired:

• If you prefer additional sweetness, add honey or maple syrup to taste.

5. Mix Well:

• Mix the ingredients well within the jar, ensuring an even distribution of oats, berries, and almond butter.

6. Refrigerate Overnight:

• Seal the jar or container and refrigerate overnight, allowing the oats and chia seeds to absorb the Liquid.

7. Top with Almonds:

• Before serving, sprinkle sliced almonds on top for a delightful crunch.

8. Garnish (Optional):

• Garnish with fresh mint leaves if desired.

9. Serve:

• Enjoy Berry Almond Overnight Oats straight from the jar or transfer them to a bowl for a delightful and nutritious breakfast.

Nutrition Information:

- Calories: 350 calories
- Protein: 15g
- Carbohydrates: 45g
- Fat: 15g
- Fiber: 10g

EDAMAME AND CARROT NOODLE STIR-FRY

Stir-Fry Description:

Experience colors, flavors, and nutrition with this Edamame and Carrot Noodle Stir-Fry. Packed with protein-rich edamame, vibrant carrot noodles, and a medley of vegetables, this stir-fry is a delicious and wholesome way to enjoy a plant-based meal.

Ingredients:

For the Stir-Fry:

• 2 cups carrot noodles (pre-spiralized or julienned)

• 1 cup edamame (fresh or frozen, thawed)

• One bell pepper (any color), thinly sliced

• One medium zucchini, spiralized or thinly sliced

• 1 cup broccoli florets

• Three green onions, sliced (white and green parts separated)

• One tablespoon of sesame oil or vegetable oil

• Sesame seeds for garnish (optional)

For the Stir-Fry Sauce:

• Three tablespoons soy sauce

• One tablespoon of hoisin sauce

• One tablespoon of rice vinegar

• One tablespoon of maple syrup or honey

• One teaspoon of grated ginger

• Two cloves garlic, minced

• One teaspoon of cornstarch mixed with two tablespoons water (cornstarch slurry)

Instructions:

1. Prepare Vegetables:

• Spiralize or julienne carrots, thinly slice bell pepper, spiralize or slice zucchini, and slice green onions.

2. Make Stir-Fry Sauce:

• Whisk together soy sauce, hoisin sauce, rice vinegar, maple syrup or honey, grated ginger, minced garlic, and cornstarch slurry in a bowl. Set aside.

3. Stir-Fry Vegetables:

• Heat sesame oil or vegetable oil in a wok or large skillet over medium-high heat.

• Add bell pepper, zucchini, broccoli, and white parts of green onions. Stir-fry for 3-4 minutes until vegetables are slightly tender.

4. Add Carrot Noodles and Edamame:

• Add carrot noodles and edamame to the wok. Stir-fry for 2-3 minutes until the carrot noodles are tender.

5. Incorporate Stir-Fry Sauce:

• Pour the prepared stir-fry sauce over the vegetables. Toss to coat evenly.

6. Cook until Sauce Thickens:

• Cook for another 2-3 minutes until the SauceSauce thickens and coats the vegetables.

7. Garnish:

• Garnish the Edamame and Carrot Noodle Stir-Fry with green parts of sliced green onions and sesame seeds if desired.

8. Serve:

• Serve hot, and enjoy this colorful and nutritious stir-fry.

Nutrition Information (per serving):

• Calories: 300 calories

• Protein: 15g

• Carbohydrates: 40g

• Fat: 10g

• Fiber: 10g

CUCUMBER AND AVOCADO GAZPACHO

Soup Description:

Cool down with the refreshing taste of Cucumber and Avocado Gazpacho. This chilled soup combines the crispness of cucumber, the creaminess of avocado, and the zing of lime for a delightful and hydrating dish, perfect for warm days or as a light appetizer.

Ingredients:

• Three cucumbers, peeled and chopped

• Two ripe avocados, peeled and diced

• 1/2 red onion, chopped

• Two cloves garlic, minced

• 1/4 cup fresh cilantro, chopped

• 1/4 cup fresh mint leaves

• One lime, juiced

• 3 cups vegetable broth, chilled

• Salt and black pepper to taste

• Extra-virgin olive oil for drizzling (optional)

• Cucumber slices and fresh herbs for garnish

Instructions:

1. Prepare Vegetables:

• Peel and chop the cucumbers, dice the avocados, chop the red onion, mince the garlic, and chop the cilantro.

2. Blend Ingredients:

• Combine chopped cucumbers, diced avocados, chopped red onion, minced garlic, cilantro, mint leaves, and lime juice in a blender.

3. Blend with Broth:

• Add chilled vegetable broth to the blender. Blend until smooth and creamy.

4. Season:

• Season the gazpacho with salt and black pepper to taste. Adjust lime juice if needed.

5. Chill:

• Transfer the gazpacho to a large bowl or individual serving bowls. Cover and refrigerate for at least 2 hours to allow the flavors to meld and the soup to chill.

6. Garnish:

• Before serving, garnish with cucumber slices, fresh herbs, and a drizzle of extra-virgin olive oil if desired.

7. Serve:

• Serve the Cucumber and Avocado Gazpacho chilled, offering your meal a refreshing and flavorful start.

Nutrition Information (per serving):

• Calories: 200 calories

- Protein: 5g
- Carbohydrates: 20g
- Fat: 15g
- Fiber: 10g

ROASTED EGGPLANT AND TOMATO CAPONATA

Caponata Description:

Indulge in the rich and savory flavors of Roasted Eggplant and Tomato Caponata. This classic Italian dish combines the earthiness of roasted eggplant, the sweetness of tomatoes, and the tanginess of capers and vinegar for a delightful appetizer or side dish.

Ingredients:

- One large eggplant, diced
- 1 pint cherry tomatoes, halved
- One onion, finely chopped
- Three cloves garlic, minced
- Two tablespoons of capers drained
- 1/4 cup Kalamata olives, pitted and chopped
- Two tablespoons of red wine vinegar
- Two tablespoons of tomato paste

- One tablespoon of honey or maple syrup

- 1/4 cup fresh basil, chopped

- Salt and black pepper to taste

- Olive oil for roasting and cooking

- Baguette slices or crackers for serving

Instructions:

1. Roast Eggplant and Tomatoes:

- Preheat the oven to 400°F (200°C).

- Place diced eggplant and halved cherry tomatoes on a baking sheet. Drizzle with olive oil, season with salt and black pepper, and toss to coat.

- Roast in the preheated oven for 25-30 minutes or until the eggplant is golden and tomatoes are blistered.

2. Sauté Onion and Garlic:

- In a large skillet, heat olive oil over medium heat. Add chopped onion and sauté until softened. Add minced garlic and cook for an additional 1-2 minutes until fragrant.

3. Combine Ingredients:

- Add the roasted eggplant and tomatoes to the skillet. Stir in capers, chopped Kalamata olives, red wine vinegar, tomato paste, and honey or maple syrup.

4. Simmer:

- Allow the mixture to simmer for 10-15 minutes, stirring occasionally, until the flavors meld and the caponata thickens.

5. Season and Finish:

• Season with salt and black pepper to taste. Stir in chopped fresh basil.

• Remove from heat and let it cool slightly.

6. Serve:

• Serve the Roasted Eggplant and Tomato Caponata warm or at room temperature with baguette slices or crackers.

Nutrition Information (per serving):

• Calories: 150 calories

• Protein: 2g

• Carbohydrates: 20g

• Fat: 8g

• Fiber: 5g

CONCLUSION

As we bid farewell to this exploration of the Myasthenia Gravis diet, let us carry forward the understanding that the journey with MG is multifaceted, and dietary choices are a dynamic part of this intricate puzzle. Collaboration with healthcare professionals, a keen awareness of individual triggers, and the cultivation of a mindful eating approach contribute to a diet that is both personalized and purposeful.

In conclusion, the Myasthenia Gravis diet embodies the spirit of resilience—an ally that supports, empowers, and nourishes. It stands as a testament to the profound connection between what we consume and how we navigate the complexities of health. May this journey into the world of MG and its dietary considerations inspire thoughtful eating and a renewed appreciation for the remarkable strength inherent in those touched by Myasthenia Gravis.